All About Join

A Maintenance Guide

DISCARD

DEMCO

ALSO BY THE AUTHOR

All About Bone: An Owner's Manual

All About Muscle: A User's Guide

The Clinical Management of Muscle Disease

Muscle and Its Diseases

First Aid Without Fear (first aid for the blind in Braille)

Posture in the Blind

The Clinical I (short stories and essays)

One Wonderful Day at a Time (juvenile)

Now and At Other Times (poetry)

101 Questions and Answers About Muscular Dystrophy

Hey, I'm Here Too! (muscle dystrophy—siblings)

101 Hints to "Help-with-Ease" for Patients with Neuromuscular Disease, A Do-It-Yourself Owner's Guide

Muscular Dystrophy in Children: A Guide for Families

All About Joints

A Maintenance Guide

Irwin M. Siegel, M.D.

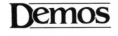

New York

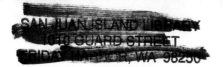
Demos Medical Publishing, Inc., 386 Park Avenue South,
New York, New York 10016

Library of Congress Cataloging-in-Publication Data

Siegel, Irwin M., 1927–
   All about joints : a maintenance guide / Irwin M. Siegel.
      p. ; cm.
   Includes bibliographical references and index.
   ISBN 1-888799-56-0 (pbk.)
   1. Joints—Diseases—Popular works.
   [DNLM: 1. Joint Diseases—Popular Works. WE 304 S571a 2002] I. Title.
   RC932 .S54 2002
   616.7'2—dc21

                                             2002000171

Made in the United States of America

Acknowledgments

I thank the following people for their assistance in the preparation of this book:

Jackie Abern, CMT, for expert transcription, grammar and syntax correction, and proofreading.

Artist Kurt Peterson for his outstanding illustrations and charts.

Patricia Casey, O.T., for reading the book and offering constructive suggestions as to content and format.

My many colleagues in the Orthopaedic department at the Rush Presbyterian–St. Luke's Medical Center and the University of Illinois for their input and support.

Karen Boone and Seena Kitchen, Department of Neurological Sciences, Rush Presbyterian–St. Luke's Medical Center, for secretarial services.

Demos Medical Publishing, of New York City, particularly President, Dr. Diana M. Schneider, and Managing Editor, Joan Wolk, for skillfully and patiently shepherding the book through editing and publication.

Without the help of the above, it would have been impossible to articulate the many pieces of *All About Joints* and fashion the book I now offer you. My gratitude to all.

"A good clinical teacher is himself a medical school."
Oliver Wendell Holmes (1809–1894)

This book is dedicated to my many teachers,
particularly the late Drs. Harold Sofield and Manley Page.

Contents

Preface xi
Foreword xiii
Introduction xv
1 Joints By and Large 1
2 Arthritis 9
3 Exercise. 31
4 The Hip 67
5 The Knee 87
6 The Ankle 105
7 The Foot 111
8 The Neck 129
9 The Spine 139
10 The Shoulder 165
11 The Elbow 177
12 The Wrist and Hand 187
13 What About the Future? 203
14 Summary. 207

15 A 12-Question Quiz to See If You Know
  All About Joints 209
  Glossary 213
  Suggestions for Further Reading 229
  Index 231

Preface

All About Joints completes a trilogy. The first volume in our musculoskeletal journey was *All About Bone* (Demos, 1998) and the second was *All About Muscle* (Demos, 2000). Each of these books was written to provide the intelligent reader with practical information about his or her bones in the first place, and muscles in the second, to enable him or her to keep these systems in the best of health. However, the ultimate dynamic purpose of bone and muscle is to create and activate joints. Hence this book, *All About Joints*—the third and final part of this musculoskeletal troika.

The purpose of this book, similar to that of its predecessors, is to inform and instruct the reader. In this case, the subject is the many important skeletal articulations that enable a child to walk, an Olympic gold medalist to excel, or a virtuoso to play the violin. Along the way, we take a look at the development, anatomy, and physiology of our joints, learning enough to enable our understanding of how they work and what we should do to keep them in shape. We survey each major joint from head to toe. Injuries and common diseases are covered, as are such important matters as diet and exercise. While reading the book, questions are encouraged, and every effort will be made to answer them.

In the past decade, modern medical science created an orthopaedic armamentarium capable of replacing almost any joint in the body. Proceeding pari passu with advances in material science and biomechanical engineering, joints are now available for the shoulder, elbow, wrist, hand, hip, knee, ankle, and foot. The cutting edge of current research deals with biological constructs such as the transplantation of cartilage into a degenerated knee. Other studies focus on artificial substitutes for bone and ligament. Arthroscopic techniques for repair of injury are now available for many joints. Imaging, including enhanced MRI and three-dimensional CT scanning, can reveal the detail of a joint's interior with noninvasive technology.

All About Joints is, of course, not only about joints because our joints, in one way or another, interface with almost every other organ system of our body. The book was written to collate and integrate much practical information, which the author hopes will be of value to anyone more than just curious about his or her body works and how to keep it working in top form.

Foreword

Irwin M. Siegel, M.D., has provided the public with yet another excellent resource to add to their knowledge of the human anatomy. In his new book, *All About Joints*, Dr. Siegel offers a concise, easy-to-understand guide to the normal and disease states of human skeletal joints. With concise, easy-to-understand language, the reader is given expert advice on the management of a wide spectrum of joint conditions running the gamut from simple sprains, osteoarthritis, and gout to the complexities of rheumatoid arthritis.

Dr. Siegel draws from his vast experience spanning over forty years as an outstanding orthopaedic surgeon in Chicago. His interest in educating the public on topics related to orthopaedics and human anatomy is most evident in his two previous books *All About Bone* (1998) and *All About Muscle* (1999). He continues to provide a service to the public with this newest praiseworthy book, *All About Joints*. Carefully written and well-illustrated, it will be another beneficial guide for the layperson who seeks to learn more about joint disorders.

Edward Abraham, M.D.
Professor and Head
Department of Orthopaedics
University of Illinois at Chicago
School of Medicine

Introduction

BONES AND JOINTS: A HISTORICAL OVERVIEW

During our lives, our bones and joints provide us with a dynamic skeleton, produce and store blood cells, hold and distribute minerals, and furnish form and support for our bodies. After we are gone, our skeletons are museums of much of what has transpired in our lives. Disease, use, and injury leave indelible marks on our bones and joints. A man buried by the eruption of Vesuvius 1,900 years ago was found with a sword by his side. His arm bones had been enlarged by years of carrying a shield in one hand and throwing a spear with the other hand. His knees were adapted to a horseman's muscles. We already knew that the Romans had a professional military, including cavalry, but if we did not, these bones would certainly bear testimony to this fact.

Harris lines, where bone is compacted similar to the lines in a tree trunk, appear in a growing bone when growth resumes after a period of malnutrition or illness. The distance from the end of the bone at the joint tells us when a Harris line was formed, and this can be correlated with the age of the individual at that time. Both chronically malnourished and well-nourished people show few Harris lines. The former rarely recover fully, and the latter have nothing from which to recover. A similar banding in tooth enamel—Wilson's bands—also reflects illness or stress in the growing years.

Wilson's bands, Harris lines, and dental caries all increase dramatically in Amer-Indians who depended heavily on maize for food as compared with other more nutritious grains. Another striking change in ancient skeletons is a general decrease in height after agriculture replaced hunter-gathering.

Study of the bones of some prehistoric Americans reveals that infant mortality was lower than in many poor, modern societies. Mortality peaked at ages 6 to 12 and 20 to 30 years. Life is apparently threatened after weaning, possibly by nutritional stress, and in early adulthood, no doubt by combat, hunting, and child-bearing. Nonetheless, many individuals survived both periods of life; skeletons have been found in England of Neanderthals, and almost 50 percent of their skulls bear marks of injury, many from stone axes. Researchers have also found well-healed fractures in chimpanzees and gorillas. When broken, bone heals with bone, not with a scar, a trait that sets it apart from almost all other body tissue.

Although the skeleton has served as a poignant reminder of death (pirates sailing under the skull and crossbones, and the dreaded Nazi SS wearing a white death's head on his uniform), bones were believed to be endowed with magical powers. In ancient Russia, burglars would fill a shin bone with marrow and hold this macabre candle aloft, circling a house in the hope of putting its inhabitants into a deathly slumber. They also carved flutes from leg bones and played them to mesmerize their marks. Some Australian aborigines severed the arm bone of their dead, in which they believed the spirit dwelled. They buried the rest of the skeleton and then, with elaborate ceremony, broke the arm bone, freeing the imprisoned spirit without incurring risk to the living or dead.

In many cultures, people have shaped bone and joint to their concept of what is beautiful. Skulls can be molded and elongated from birth, as was done by the Chinook Indian tribe of the Pacific Northwest. Such a sculptured skull was a mark of nobility, serving as a sign of elevated social rank. Although seldom practiced today, this custom has its modern equivalent in fancy hairstyling. The Chinese custom of binding women's feet, prized for its erotic appeal, provided dainty feet and a mincing step, but crippled the women treated in this way. The Chinese "lotus foot" has its contemporary counterpart in ultra-high-heeled shoes.

Old English folk tales relate that, in punishment for the twelfth century murder of Thomas à Becket, the Archbishop of Canterbury, the people of Kent were cursed to be born with tails, a sign of kinship with the devil. Every human being does, in fact, have the vestige of a tail. It is tucked under the sacrum (sacred bone), with which it articulates through a small joint, and called the coccyx (cuckoo = "bill"). The coccyx is composed of four fused vertebrae and is the only portion of the spinal column without a function. It can be bruised or broken during a fall and sometimes has to be removed because of persistent pain at the sacrococcygeal joint.

Ancient treatment for bone and joint injury began on the battlefield. In *The Iliad*, Homer describes 147 wounds, often in precise clinical language. *The Smith Papyrus*, composed about 1650 B.C., is one of the first known medical texts. It contains information on how to treat 48 wounds and injuries to bones and joints. It is thought to express the wisdom of Imhotep, a physician who learned his art healing workers injured building the Pyramids he designed.

A professor of medicine in Paris, Nicholas André, coined the term *orthopaedics* from the Greek word "orthos" (straight) and "paidios" (child). André spent his career devising means to correct bone and joint deformity.

The largest animal ever to live, the blue whale, can weigh up to 150 tons. Nonetheless, it moves with the grace of a feather floating on air because the ocean buoys its weight by meeting it with equal force to provide external support. But out of water, large animals such as dinosaurs rely solely on their skeletons for support. Like their cousins who live in the sea, birds (the direct descendants of dinosaurs) and mammals must conquer the force of gravity. The bones and joints of the bird are designed for flight, being as light and streamlined as possible. The elephant, the largest of land animals, can reach a weight of eight tons. To sustain its weight, an elephant's bones are as sturdy as tree trunks. By contrast, the femur, the longest and strongest of human bones, can resist a compressive force of 1,200 pounds per cubic inch when we walk. Although bone has the power to remodel and reshape itself under stress, it will break when tension exceeds 10 tons per square inch.

Bone derives its strength by weaving protein and mineral into a resilient fabric. Ninety-nine percent of the calcium and 85 percent of all the phosphorus in the body is found in the bones. An elastic protein called *collagen* is ounce-for-ounce stronger than steel when blended with bony crystals. After the minerals in the bone are removed, the bone becomes so rubbery that it can be tied into a knot like a garden hose. Try placing a chicken bone in a jar of vinegar. The acetic acid will leach out the minerals, leaving a bone that can be bent and twisted like a string. Scientists believe that the mineral crystals somehow seal the bone, protecting collagen from decomposition. A close artificial analogue to bone is fiberglass, which is made of slender glass threads embedded in epoxy.

Bone is the only tissue containing cells that destroy its structure (osteoclasts = Gr. bone, to break) as well as cells that build it up (osteoblasts = Gr. bone, germ). Throughout life, bone regenerates and repairs itself through an endocrine-driven system. Any disruption of this process can lead to a variety of metabolic bone diseases, including osteoporosis, rheumatoid arthritis, Paget's disease, and periodontal pathology.

In addition to providing support, small piezoelectric currents are transmitted in bones at points of compression. Bone may act as a kind of generator, translating mechanical forces into electrical response. Utilizing this knowledge, devices that generate magnetic currents are used to speed healing in broken bones and joints.

Although ancient bones and joints have provided information regarding our planet, the prehistory of the Earth, as well as human ancestry, it is a good thing that bones and joints do eventually decompose. It has been estimated that the total weight of all living things that have ever inhabited the Earth equals the weight of the planet itself! If bones did not decompose, every square foot of dry land would be piled yards high in skeletal remains.

Leonardo Da Vinci's experience in engineering led him to consider the skeleton as a set of rigid levers. From his understanding of the function of muscles, da Vinci deduced the operation of these levers. This genius of the Renaissance created models of joints to gain a deeper understanding of their function.

The skeleton's most important role is that of support. However, *articulations* are necessary to orchestrate movement. For example, consider the adult spine, engineered for both strength and flexibility. Its 33 vertebrae, separated by flexible discs, are gracefully curved to facilitate the upright posture. These vertebrae have become specialized, with differences dictated by requirements for movement. The adult spinal discs absorb shock and allow motion between the vertebrae. The spinal column crosses the line of gravity, its curve providing more stability and strength than if the spine were straight. The spine has adapted to our erect stance, allowing us to walk on two feet, freeing our hands for tasks more complicated than bearing weight. Anthropologists believe that bipedalism (two-legged walking) has led to an increase in the size of the human brain.

With this brief overview of some of the history of bones and joints, we begin our review of the wonderful skeletal structures that distinguish us from lower life forms and enable us to experience the joys and rewards of highly controlled movement.

All About Joints

A Maintenance Guide

1

Joints By and Large

"This frame, compacted with transcendent skill,
of moving joints, obedient to my will . . ."

John Arbuthnot
Know Yourself

The need for strength requires bones to be rigid. However, movement would be almost impossible if our skeletons were solid bone. Nature has solved this problem in vertebrates, including humans, by casting the skeleton into many bones and creating joints where they intersect. Joints are custom-formed to serve the functional needs of the limbs that contain them. They are held together by fibrous tissue (capsule and ligaments) and continuously lubricated to offset friction. In this way joints permit motion, which grants us humans a much more complex repertoire of movement than, say, most insects, spiders, and crustaceans, which, like the joints in your fingers, move only in one plane. However, we are not quite as versatile as invertebrates and certain millipedes, which can rotate one skeletal ring upon the next, curving their axis in any direction, even walking with their legs on the ground at a right angle to their coiled position.

The words *articulation* (L. articulatio—the junction between bones) and *joint* (L. junctio—a joining or connection) are used synonymously to refer to those structural arrangements that connect two or more bones. Although most joints permit at least some movement between the bones they connect, this is not essential for a connecting structure to be called a joint. The function of some joints is to allow the joined

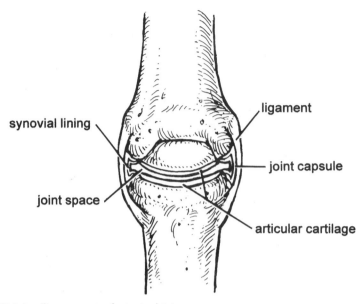

FIGURE 1-1   Components of a typical joint.

structures to grow until they in turn become as solid as the bones they connect.

Where joints are immovable, as in the articulations between the bones of the growing skull, the adjacent margins of the bone are separated merely by a thin layer of fibrous tissue. Where slight movement but great strength is required, the joint surfaces are united by tough elastic fibrocartilages, as in the joints between the vertebral bodies. In freely movable joints, such as the shoulder or knee, the surfaces are completely separated and the bones expanded for greater convenience of mutual connection. They are covered by *cartilage* and enveloped by fibrous tissue capsules.

ARTICULAR CARTILAGE

Articular cartilage is of a type called *hyaline* (glasslike) cartilage because thin sections of it are translucent or even transparent to light. In contrast to bone, it is easily cut. It is deformable under pressure, but elastic so that it quickly recovers its shape. These properties are important for its function under conditions of *loading* (bearing weight). A membrane lines the interior of such joints.

This *synovial* (Gr. syn.—together; L. ovum—egg) membrane secretes a thick viscous liquid that lubricates the joint. It also regulates protein and electrolyte (ionic or electrically charged molecule) metabolism in the joint and removes waste from the joint.

Joints are strengthened by *ligaments*, strong fibrous bands that connect the bones that form the joint (Fig 1.1).

DEVELOPMENT

Bone and joint both develop from the middle layer of tissue in the embryo. Circumscribed condensation of cells in this mesoderm (middle skin) become chondrified (turned into cartilage) and finally ossified (turned into bone) to form the bones of the skeleton. The intervening noncondensed portions of tissue develop into joints.

As soon as the joint cavity appears during development, it contains watery fluid. The tissue surrounding the original mesodermal cellular core forms fibrous sheaths for the developing bones, which continue between their ends as the capsules of the joints. Ligaments develop both in these capsules and as derivations from tendons surrounding the joint. After the joint cavity is established during the third month of gestation, the muscles that move the joint begin to contract. This movement enhances nutrition of the articular cartilage and prevents fusion of the apposed joint surfaces. Early restriction of joint motion can result in permanent loss of the joint cavity, whereas later restriction can lead to abnormalities of the soft tissues associated with the joint. Because normal positioning of the fetus in the uterus permits a fair degree of movement of the upper limbs but restricts the legs—which are folded and pressed firmly against the body—the lower limbs are more vulnerable to *congenital* (found at birth) joint deformity such as clubfoot or congenital hip dislocation. In several of the movable joints, a portion of the mesodermal tissue that originally existed between the ends of the bones persists and forms an *articular disc*. An example of this is the *menisci* (cartilages) of the knee joint.

TYPES OF JOINTS

There are various types of joints. The skull type is immovable, the vertebral type is slightly movable, and the limb type is freely movable. Joints of the skull are temporary until they fuse, those of the vertebrae are secure, and limb type joints or synovial articulations, although freely movable, are insecure. Immovable joints are called *synarthroses*, slightly movable joints are labeled *amphiarthroses*, and freely movable joints are called *diarthroses*.

The greatest number of joints in the body are diarthroses. Varieties of these joints have been determined by the kind of motion each allows. Joints permit:

- ❑ *gliding* movement
- ❑ *flexion*, where the angle between adjoining bones is decreased, as when the forearm is moved forward and upward
- ❑ *extension*, where the angle between adjoining bones is increased, as when the forearm is straightened
- ❑ *abduction*, when an extremity is moved away from the body or adduction, when an arm or leg is moved toward the body
- ❑ *circumduction* (circular movement), best seen in ball-and-socket joints
- ❑ *rotation*, where a bone moves around a central axis without undergoing any displacement.

Some examples of *hinge joints* are the elbow and the knee; *ball-and-socket joints*, the shoulder and hip; *gliding joints*, the small bones of the foot and the wrist, the ribs, and the vertebrae. A *saddle joint*, which permits movement in two directions, unites the thumb with the hand.

MECHANICS

Bones in a freely movable joint articulate in pairs, each pair distinguished by its own pair of conarticular surfaces. These surfaces constitute "mating pairs." Each mating pair consists of a "male" surface and a "female" surface. Following an engineering convention, a joint surface is called male if it is convex and female if it is concave.

In all positions of a diarthrosis—except one—the conarticular surfaces fit imperfectly. Such incongruence is not great and

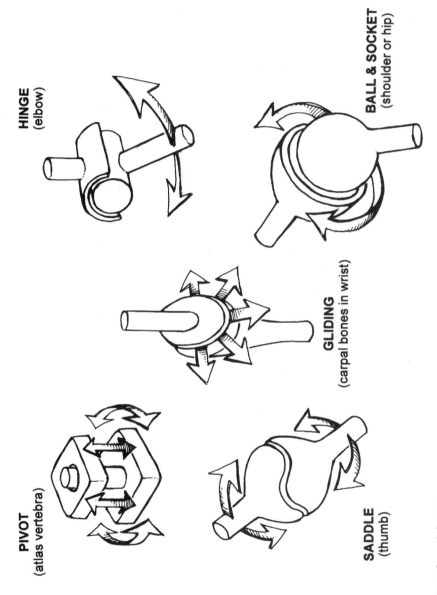

HINGE
(elbow)

BALL & SOCKET
(shoulder or hip)

GLIDING
(carpal bones in wrist)

PIVOT
(atlas vertebra)

SADDLE
(thumb)

FIGURE 1-2 Some joint types.

is lessened by mutual alteration of the opposed parts of the surfaces. This is a consequence of the plasticity of hyaline cartilage.

The exceptional position is called the *close-packed* position,
in which the entire articulating portion of the female surface is
in complete contact with the apposed male surface. Functionally,
this changes the joint from a freely movable joint to a "locked"
one, and it is the position in which the joint is most stable.

Every joint has its close-packed position. A good example is
the wrist when the hand is fully bent backward (dorsiflexed) on
the forearm. Another is the knee when the thigh and leg are in
the military position of attention.

The close-packed position is not assumed often or constantly because it requires special muscular effort. It is also dangerous because two bones in series are converted temporarily into
a functionally single but longer unit that is more likely to be
injured by sudden stress. For example, sprain or even fracture
of an ankle occurs when that joint, close-packed, is suddenly and
violently bent.

SYNOVIAL JOINTS

Synovial joints, which allow free movement, must have their surfaces lubricated. The lubricant is called *synovial fluid* because it
has the consistency of egg white. Although synovial fluid is 95 percent water, it enables the cartilaginous joint surfaces to move with
less friction than that of ice sliding on ice. Synovial fluid (like
printer's ink and certain gels) has the unusual ability to become
thick or thin with change of pressure, a property called *thixotropy*.

FAT PADS

Some of the larger joints contain *fat pads*. The function of these
structures depends on the fact that fat is liquid in the living
body and therefore easily deformable. These fat pads contribute
to the "internal streamlining" of the joint cavity, preventing
eddying (whiplash motion) of the synovial fluid. Their deforma-
bility enables them to do this effectively.

In addition, the fat pads keep the synovial fluid sufficiently
thin between the neighboring parts of the male and female sur-

faces, with proper elasticity as well as viscosity, to effectively lubricate the joint.

A fat pad can be pinched as a result of an accident. This is very painful because of the large number of pain nerve fibers found in these pads.

All About Joints will describe every major joint in your body from the top of your head to the tips of your toes. We will present the anatomy of each joint and discuss how it works. We will talk about injury and disease, diagnosis, and treatment. When considering joints and their diseases, exercise is important, and we will discuss this in some detail. State-of-the-art research into the newest therapies will be presented. Illustrative case reports will be outlined. At the end of each chapter queries and answers concerning the joint in question will be presented. A glossary, review, and suggestions for further reading are appended at the end of the book.

But before we look at your joints one by one, let's first talk about the bane of all joints, arthritis.

2

Arthritis

"When your joints, instead of your breakfast cereal,
go snap, crackle and pop, you know you're over the hill."

Anonymous

Bone is a "user-friendly" bodily system. It repairs, adapts, and remodels easily. Nonetheless, it ages like the rest of the body, and arthritis usually cannot be avoided, at least not the "normal" aging degeneration found in joints. However, something *can* be done about this condition. This chapter offers a general survey of arthritis and tells you how it is treated. The management of arthritic problems concerned with each specific joint has been covered in detail in the chapter on that joint.

CARTILAGE

Our joints permit movement, but in doing so they are often subjected to considerable stress and strain. Joints are lined with hyaline (glasslike) cartilage (L.—gristle). Cartilage is composed mainly of a protein called collagen, which is embedded in a firm gel, and is thus more flexible than bone and uniquely structured to withstand tremendous abuse. It can resist crushing by loads considerably greater than those required to break a bone. Articular cartilage has a capacity for repair and regeneration in response to normal wear and tear, but cartilage lacks blood vessels and is nourished only by diffusion of nutrients from the fluid found in the joints.

The cells that form connective tissue during embryonic development have the potential to differentiate along several lines (fibrous tissue, cartilage, or bone), depending on local conditions, which include pressure. Rays and sharks are good examples of mechanical engineering efficiency. Their anatomical perseverance from the Devonian era (375 million years ago) attests to the suitability of their nonbony, cartilaginous endoskeleton. Rays and sharks do not develop arthritis because they do not have bones.

Joints are lubricated either by "weeping lubrication," in which the synovial fluid absorbed by the cartilage is squeezed out when the joint surface is pressed, or by "boosted lubrication," in which the articular cartilage absorbs some molecules of the synovial fluid, allowing molecular mucous compounds to remain behind to lubricate the joint.

SOME GENERAL REMARKS

The word *arthritis* means inflammation of a joint (arthr = joint; itis = inflammation). The signs of arthritis have been identified in the bones of dinosaurs as well as those of contemporary mammals.

There are more than 100 different forms of arthritis. As many as 40 million people in the United States have one type or another, with a projected prevalence of 60 million by the year 2020. Arthritis is a serious illness for many people and a major cause of absence from work. Degenerative arthritis of the knee alone accounts for as much impairment in older Americans as conditions such as diabetes, heart disease, hip fracture, and depression. It is a major reason for lost time at work and causes significant disability, resulting in the hospitalization of more than 50,000 people each year. Although arthritis is mainly a disease of adults, there are childhood forms; arthritis affects 250,000 young people under 16 years of age in the United States alone.

INFLAMMATION

Inflammation is one of the body's normal reactions to disease or injury and represents the body's natural defenses at work. In a diseased or injured joint, inflammation results in stiffness, pain, and swelling. Although usually temporary, inflammation can cause permanent damage in arthritic joints. At the same time, arthritis can be primarily infectious because of a variety of bacterial agents, including gonorrhea and tuberculosis, or even viral (e.g., German measles, smallpox). Parasitic infections are unusual, but cases of joint involvement by the guinea worm, a nematode that affects 50 million people in tropical countries, have been documented. Destructive changes and deformities of the joints can occur in leprosy (Hansen's disease). These arise from infections of the nerves. A chronic rheumatoid-like arthritis in swine has for many years been a major cause for the rejection of pork in the United States and other countries. *Mycoplasma* organisms are minute bacteria that cause arthritis in many bird and mammalian species.

SOFT TISSUES

Certain conditions of the *soft tissues*—ligaments, fascia, tendons, and bursae—are "cousins" of arthritis that frequently mimic it. Such disorders fall under the general rubric of *soft tissue rheumatism* (from the Greek word *rheumatismos*, meaning suffering from a flux). They can affect young as well as older individuals, and it has been estimated that there are 12 million such people in the United States alone.

Some of the disorders in this group of soft tissue diseases are tendinitis, capsulitis, bursitis, fasciitis, ligamentitis, and fibrositis. Inflammation of the soft tissues can occur as the result of an infection or excessive use of the part involved. The names given to these painful conditions reflect the many occupations, sports, and recreations that are affected. Consider ballet toe, dancer's hip, golfer's elbow, housemaid's or jumper's knee, Pac-man tendinitis, tennis elbow, marcher's heel, bowler's thumb, weaver's bottom, and the like.

Cartilage in locations other than a joint (for instance, between the ribs and the sternum) can also become inflamed, mimicking arthritis. Muscles can also be irritated and painful. This is called *myositis* or *myalgia* (myo = muscular; algia = pain) as part of an arthritic condition or in isolation, leading to symptoms that may be confused with arthritis. Because pain is the "alarm system" of the body, it is important to make as exact a diagnosis as possible and not just "take something for the pain." If arthritic-like pain does not respond to over-the-counter medication and home remedies within a reasonable period of time, a doctor should be consulted.

OTHER TYPES OF ARTHRITIS

Because of the close connection between the *psyche* (mind) and the *soma* (body), arthritic and nonarthritic pain can be exaggerated or even caused by an agitated mental state. When there is no organic cause of pain and disability, the condition is called psychogenic rheumatism.

Ankylosing spondylitis is an inflammation in which the soft tissues attach to bone. It most commonly affects the spine, stiffening and eventually fusing it. It also affects the hips. Ankylosing spondylitis tends to run in families because of the inheritance of a specific gene. The disease affected the Florentine ruler Cosimo de Medici and the French poet Paul Scarron.

Polymyalgia rheumatica is a condition of stiffness in the neck, shoulders, and hips that is often seen in older women. Pains around the joints occur and can mimic those of arthritis. A particular blood test, the *sedimentation rate* (a measure of bodily inflammation), is always elevated in this condition. In some cases polymyalgia rheumatica is a manifestation of an underlying inflammatory blood vessel disease called *giant cell arteritis*, which can affect the temporal (forehead) arteries, causing headache, visceral disturbance, and severe jaw pain (claudication). Treatment is with low doses of corticosteroid drugs. Therapy must be continued for a long period of time, as the steroids are gradually reduced. It is very dangerous to stop taking steroid medication abruptly, because the body's ability to produce its own steroids is depressed while taking steroids by mouth and is only gradually reestablished as the oral medication is slowly withdrawn.

Now let's consider the most familiar forms of arthritis—osteoarthritis, rheumatoid arthritis, and gout (Figure 2-1).

OSTEOARTHRITIS

Sometimes called *degenerative* arthritis, this condition of wear and tear in the joints is the most common form of arthritis. All

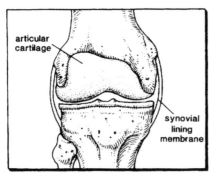

A healthy knee joint.

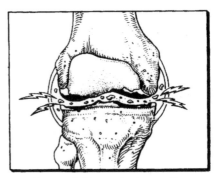

Osteoarthritis—articular cartilge degenerates and fragments.

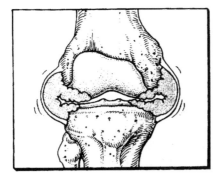

Rheumatoid arthritis—an inflamed synovial membrane erodes the joint.

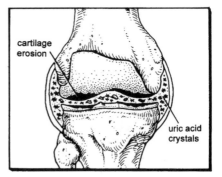

Gouty arthritis—cartilage erosion with uric acid crystals found in the joint.

FIGURE 2-1   The arthritis scenario.

adults past middle age are affected to some degree. Many historical figures suffered from severe osteoarthritis, including the emperor Constantine, Mary Queen of Scots, and James Madison. Grandma Moses, a notable American folk artist, only began to paint seriously in her later years (she lived to be 101) after her children had grown and left home and osteoarthritis of her hands prevented her from sewing and doing needlework.

It is estimated that 17 million people in the United States have osteoarthritis. It is caused by the breakdown of the articular cartilage inside a joint. The cartilage loses its ability to act as a "shock absorber," and little "spurs" form at the margins of the joint. Although osteoarthritis occurs as a natural consequence of aging, it may begin earlier as a result of joint overuse or an injury such as a fracture or repeated sprain. Certain diseases such as hypothyroidism or diabetes predispose one to osteoarthritis. Congenital and hereditary diseases, such as congenital dislocation of the hip, can also bring about secondary osteoarthritis. Major weight-bearing joints other than the hip can be involved. This includes the spine and knees.

Osteonecrosis of the knee can mimic osteoarthritis. Osteonecrosis is a sudden collapse of one of the articular surfaces of the femur at the knee joint that occurs in older people; its cause is not known. Treatment is surgery either to realign the knee to shift weight off the collapsed bone or to replace the damaged bone with a prosthetic joint. The shoulders, wrists, and elbows occasionally are affected, particularly if these joints have been overused or injured.

Nearly 90 percent of all people over the age of 60 show some signs of osteoarthritis. Although there is no cure, relief may be obtained through the use of drugs, physical therapy, and surgery in selected cases.

Osteoarthritis may be caused or accelerated by malalignment of weight-bearing joints. It appears to have a hereditary basis. Osteoarthritis is found in other diseases such as *acromegaly*, in which an excess of growth hormone causes bony overgrowth and arthritis. The character "Jaws" in the James Bond movies displays such features.

Normally smooth cartilage becomes irregular, restricting motion and causing pain on movement. Knobby points of cartilage and bone may develop at the ends of the fingers (Heberden's nodes) or at the middle of the fingers (Bouchard's nodes). As the cartilage breaks down, localized inflammation with spillage of irritating chemicals into the joint can cause pain. Erosion of cartilage then proceeds to expose underlying bone, which results in more inflammation, pain, and stiffness. Muscles go into spasm and become fatigued. In the lower back, breakdown of the intervertebral disc may cause pain, and overgrowth of bone can result in pressure on spinal nerves, leading to *sciatica*. Osteoarthritis of the neck may similarly cause nerve root pressure, with pain spreading to the ear or shoulder. Hip pain can radiate to the buttocks or groin, and knee instability and weakness can cause difficulty, particularly when walking stairs. People with osteoarthritis usually find that stiffness is worse after rest and that their joints loosen up with activity, although some people find that stiffness and pain increase as the day goes on. Creaking or grating sounds (crepitus) in the joints may be experienced on movement.

Patients with suspected osteoarthritis require a complete medical workup that includes a history and physical examination, X-rays, and occasionally aspiration of joint fluid. Blood tests can rule out other types of arthritis, such as gouty arthritis and rheumatoid arthritis. The blood from patients who have gout contains an overabundance of uric acid, and the blood from a patient with rheumatoid arthritis often reveals a specific rheumatoid factor. Other blood examinations include DNA or antinuclear tests. X-rays in osteoarthritis show joint narrowing caused by cartilage loss as well as bony overgrowth with thickening of the bones about the involved joints. There may be an excess of synovial fluid in response to joint irritation.

Treatment

A variety of drugs are available to treat the pain of osteoarthritis. Aspirin is a time-proven anodyne (anti-pain) and anti-inflammatory drug. A precursor of aspirin, salicin, found in the bitter leaves of the willow tree, was known to Hippocrates. Aspirin was discovered in 1889 and became available over-the-counter circa 1900. Americans use approximately 175 aspirin tablets per person each year. This amounts to 80 million aspirin a day or 16,000 tons of aspirin each year for the country as a whole. Aspirin is usually taken with food and/or antacids to minimize stomach upset. Those allergic to aspirin may develop an asthmatic reaction that involves wheezing or shortness of breath. Aspirin decreases the ability of blood to clot (that is why it is administered to prevent heart attacks). Large doses can cause tinnitus (ringing in the ears). Enteric-coated aspirin should not irritate the stomach. It should not be given with milk, however, because milk quickly dissolves the coating. Aspirin should never be taken with either alcohol or vitamin C; such combinations may seriously irritate the gastrointestinal (GI) tract.

Nonsteroidal antiinflammatory drugs (NSAIDs) are a class of drugs available for the treatment of osteoarthritis. More than 60 million prescriptions for NSAIDs are written each year, and 30 million over-the-counter pills are sold annually in the United

States. Although they are often effective, these drugs may have side effects that include stomach upset and kidney or liver damage. Anyone taking an NSAID should be closely monitored by his or her physician.

Aspirin is technically an NSAID. Examples of other drugs in this category include piroxicam (Feldene), diclofenate sodium (Voltaren), ibuprofen (Motrin), indomethacin (Indocin), naproxen (Naprosyn), sulindac (Clinoril), tolmetin (Tolectin), diflunisal (Dolobid), oxaprozin (Daypro), and nabumetone (Relafen). Ibuprofen has been available over-the-counter since 1984, and naproxen has been available since 1994. The sales of over-the-counter pain relievers last year was $26.67 billion.

So-called COX-2 inhibitors selectively block cyclooxygenase-2, an enzyme that produces *prostaglandins*, chemicals responsible for the pain and swelling that accompany arthritis. Traditional NSAIDs relieve pain by blocking COX-2, but they also block COX-1, an enzyme that protects the lining of the stomach and duodenum. A 1998 study attributed 16,500 deaths yearly in the United States to stomach perforations, ulcers, and bleeds resulting from the chronic use of NSAIDs. Thus, the newer COX-2 inhibitors such as celecoxib (Celebrex) and rofecoxib (Vioxx), which do not block COX-1, are strong performers in the arthritis pain medication field because they are perceived to fill an unmet need for an anti-inflammatory medication as or more potent than existing NSAID drugs but with fewer GI side effects. Although better than other NSAIDs, COX-2 inhibitors are not completely safe. They still can irritate the GI tract.

Another problem with COX-2 inhibitors is that whereas traditional NSAIDs can cost as little as 20 cents a pill, the new COX-2 inhibitors cost about 15 times as much. Much less expensive than either is macrodosing with vitamins C, D, and E, which has been shown to be beneficial in slowing the progression of osteoarthritis of the knee. Vitamin C is believed to have many beneficial effects beyond those of an antioxidant. It appears to be involved in protein construction and especially the synthesis of collagen, which is essential to the development of cartilage. Therefore, vitamin C may aid cartilage repair following an injury.

Corticosteroids are often useful when they are injected directly into an osteoarthritic joint. The joint is first *aspirated* (fluid is withdrawn) and the steroid is then injected. This can markedly decrease inflammation and pain in joints. However, corticosteroids should not be used indiscriminately or over a long period of time because of side effects that may include fluid retention, increased blood pressure, osteoporosis, gastrointestinal bleeding, weight gain, fat distribution changes, proneness to infections, slow healing of injuries, and cataracts, to mention but a few.

Muscle relaxants are sometimes used to decrease muscle spasm. Various liniments that act as counterirritants producing local heat may give temporary relief of pain. Capsaicin cream, a nonprescription drug derived from the pepper plant, can provide analgesia by inhibiting chemical pain transmission.

A combination of glucosamine and chondroitin sulfate seems to work to build damaged joint tissues in osteoarthritis. For several years, veterinarians have used a version of glucosamine (glucosamine sulfate) to treat osteoarthritis in animals. The effectiveness of these supplements in humans is now under study.

Injecting sodium hyaluronate (Hyalgan) or a similar substance directly into the joint provides relief of osteoarthritis in selected cases. This treatment is called *viscosupplementation* because it provides a gel-like "padding" within the joint that relieves pressure and pain. However, there can be significant side effects including an acute inflammatory reaction to the injection.

Excessive weight gain places undue stress on arthritic joints, and the person with osteoarthritis must keep slim if possible. At the same time he or she should maintain general nutrition with a well-balanced, vitamin-supplemented diet. Involved joints may be protected with splints, and walking aids such as canes and crutches can be used. Every five pounds of pressure applied to a cane relieves the supporting leg of 25 pounds of load. Activities of daily living should be performed in the least stressful manner. Devices such as wall brackets in the tub or a raised toilet seat can make day-to-day living more comfortable.

Exercise is excellent treatment for arthritis as it keeps joints well-lubricated and mobile. Exercise should be supervised by a physical therapist, who can design a program that will increase the range of motion of involved joints, amplify strength, and improve function. Resistance exercises and even aerobic exercise can strengthen muscles so that they are better able to protect joints by absorbing shock and improving stability. Exercise also increases joint flexibility, which lessens pain and decreases the risk of sprains. The joint pressure that occurs with exercise helps cartilage squeeze out waste and soak up nutrients and oxygen. The more a joint is exercised, the healthier it is likely to be.

Moist heat often alleviates chronic discomfort, and cold packs may be used for acute distress. The pain and stiffness of osteoarthritic hands can be relieved by warm wax treatments. Ultrasound and even diathermy have been used with success. Transcutaneous electrical nerve stimulation (TENS) consists of a portable battery wired to pads that attach to the skin. The electrical current stimulates nerves, thereby relieving pain.

Alternative therapies include acupuncture, which increases the production of *endorphins* (the body's natural painkillers), provides counterirritation, and closes a selected central nervous system "gate" to pain. The use of magnets is another option. This has received new-found attention from such sports stars as Dan Marino, Andre Agassi, and Hideki Irabu. Magnet therapy is an ancient medical tradition and a commonly accepted practice outside the United States, especially in Eastern cultures that believe that the life force is magnetic energy. Magnetic therapy is noninvasive, is relatively inexpensive, and apparently has no serious side effects. The basic premise is that a magnetic force applied to the body expands blood vessels and increases blood flow. Research has shown that this increased circulation can accelerate healing and reduce pain. The exact means by which magnets achieve their results is really not known; it is mostly speculation. Physicians who use magnetotherapy in their practice claim that, like vitamins and sunlight, the body simply needs a certain amount of magnetic energy to function. Several recent studies have shown positive results with the use of magnets in treating arthritis. U.S. consumers will spend more than $500 million this year on magnetic pads, bracelets, back wraps, and seat cushions. Other products available include magnetic insoles, wraps (for ankles, knees, the back, elbows, shoulders, and the neck) and even mattresses and pillow pads to relieve pain and increase circulation during sleep. Most of these appliances can be obtained over-the-counter at your local drugstore. The treatment is relatively inexpensive. Magnetic back belts can be purchased for less than $60, insoles for approximately $40, and individual magnets for as little as $19.95, and the magnets never wear out. According to a 1998 report, the percentage of users receiving insurance coverage for "energy healing" rose from 0 percent in 1990 to 30.8 percent in 1997. The most frequently cited energy healing technique involved the use of magnets.

The main charge leveled against magnet therapy is that it is *palliative* rather than *curative*. Advocates say that, although magnets do not heal, they allow the body to do what it does better. Some practitioners are concerned that magnet therapy is being used instead of necessary medical intervention. The danger of using magnet therapy in lieu of informed medical care is compounded by the way in which magnetic devices are currently being marketed. For the most part they are sold directly to the consumer. You can search the Internet and find thousands of references to magnetic therapy, most advertising a wide range of biomagnetic devices. Contraindications for using magnet therapy include patients with pacemakers, pregnant women, and those with surgically implanted metal clips or metal parts in the area where the magnet is applied. Although magnets appear to be safe and effective, more work must be done before they become part of mainstream medicine, and the question still remains whether the use of magnets can reach harmful exposure levels.

Every year Americans spend almost $1 billion on unproved arthritis medicines. Many of these are dietary supplements that are not required to undergo the rigorous testing or federal regulation that a drug must go through before the U.S. Food and Drug Administration allows it on the market. Some of the latest fads include herbal medications. These are harmless in many cases, but some combinations can have serious side effects when they are taken without supervision.

Finally, surgery may be beneficial for osteoarthritic pain that does not respond to conventional therapy. Surgical procedures include tidal irrigation (joint flushing); realignment of the involved joint (now possible with computer assistance to plan and help perform the surgery with three-dimensional accuracy); total joint replacement of the hip, knee, finger, toe, wrist, elbow, shoulder, or ankle; fusion, which permanently holds the bone ends together preventing motion with attendant pain; or arthroscopic *debridement*, a sort of "housecleaning" of the affected joint.

Several methods to stimulate the growth of new articular cartilage in the area of denuded bone, usually in the knees, are under current investigation. One of these involves abrasion or microfracture of the bony surfaces. This stimulates the production of cartilage during healing. Another is the reimplantation of *chondrocytes* (cartilage cells) that have been harvested from elsewhere in the body and expanded in culture. Finally, there is arthroscopic *osteochondral grafting*, described as "stealing little pieces of good articular cartilage, putting them where the problem is, and holding them in place." Cartilage can be taken from the patient (autograft) or from a bone bank (allograft). Preliminary results using this technique seem promising for the treatment of osteoarthritic defects of the elbow, ankle, and knee.

CASE REPORT—OSTEOARTHRITIS

Sylvia M., a 66-year-old homemaker and mother of three grown children, experienced increasing stiffness in her knees and hips after rest. As the day wore on, she had to sit frequently to relieve pain in these joints. The last joints of several of her fingers were developing tender swellings that were firm to the touch. Sylvia had been an active person all her life and was a recreational athlete (golfing and swimming), but now pain was even preventing her from accompanying her husband on the long walks they so much enjoyed.

Sylvia attempted to treat her condition with over-the-counter medications and frequent rest. This provided minimal relief, so she consulted her doctor. A thorough history was taken and a physical examination was performed. Sylvia's doctor ordered X-rays of her hips, knees, and hands. Findings consistent with osteoarthritis were revealed. Blood tests failed to show any evidence of rheumatoid arthritis, infection, or other articular (joint) disease.

A prescription NSAID was recommended and Sylvia was advised to take off 10 pounds because she was a bit overweight. Physical therapy treatments were prescribed, including warm whirlpool baths for Sylvia's hips and knees as well as a supervised program of exercise. She was encouraged to continue with her swimming but to use a cane for long-distance walking. If this conservative program of management is not successful, Sylvia may require injections of cortisone into any joint that is symptomatic. Her osteoarthritis will be monitored closely. Severe joint destruction in the future could require joint replacement surgery.

RHEUMATOID ARTHRITIS

Rheumatoid or inflammatory arthritis is the second most common form of arthritis. It affects approximately 7 million Americans. Rheumatoid arthritis has had some famous sufferers, among the most notable being the classical artist Peter Paul Rubens and the Impressionist painters Renoir, Dufy, and Matisse, whose severe arthritic hand deformities strongly influenced the work of their later years. These artists favored bright and clear colored paints based on toxic heavy metals and fewer earth colors containing harmless carbon and iron compounds. Heavy exposure to mercury sulfide, cadmium sulfide, arsenic sulfide, lead, tin, cobalt, antimony, chromium, and manganese—the metals of the colors they preferred—may have contributed to the development of their inflammatory rheumatism. Artists today are not so exposed, but heavy metal contamination in food and drinking water still exists.

The hand deformities of rheumatoid arthritis have been depicted in classical paintings of the Flemish-Dutch school (Escorial Museum near Madrid, Spain); in Corot's *Gipsy Girl with Mandolin* (1870–1875) (National Gallery of Art, Washington, D.C.), and by the American artist Andrew Wyeth in his painting *Christina's World* (1948).

Rheumatoid arthritis initially involves the synovial membrane and is characterized by a *chronic* (long-lasting) inflammatory disease of joints and other parts of the body such as the heart and the lungs. In rheumatoid arthritis the joint fluid contains erosive chemicals that attack and corrode the joint surface. These chemicals are produced by the joint lining, which swells and thickens, eroding and severely damaging the articular cartilage. The inflamed synovial membrane that swells into the joint is called a *pannus* (L. piece of cloth). The joints most commonly affected in rheumatoid arthritis are the hands (particularly the first joints of the fingers, which develop a spindle-shaped enlargement), wrists, feet, and ankles, although large weight-bearing joints such as the hips and knees may also be involved. Swelling, pain, stiffness, and deformity are usually present. Multiple joints may be affected simultaneously, although there are cases in which only one or two joints are involved. The juvenile form of rheumatoid arthritis (Still's disease) can be crippling.

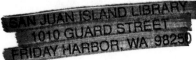

The cause of rheumatoid arthritis is not known, although it is believed to be an *autoimmune* disease. This is a condition in which the involved body tissue, in this case the synovial lining of the joints, is the victim of an immune response against itself.

Rheumatoid arthritis can affect anyone. More than 70 percent of people with this disease are over 30 years of age, and most are women. It usually affects those who have a fair complexion and red hair. A history of joint stiffness, swelling, and progressive limitation of motion is common. Physical examination reveals tenderness and swelling about the joints, especially those of the midportion of the fingers. Soft tissue rheumatoid nodules may appear around joints, particularly the elbow.

Laboratory Tests

Mild anemia is present and the sedimentation rate may be elevated. Special blood tests for rheumatoid arthritis include those for "rheumatoid factors." X-rays early in the course of the disease show only thinning (osteopenia) of the bone around involved joints, but severe degenerative changes can be seen as the inflammatory process progresses. Joint aspiration reveals inflammation of joint fluid, with cloudiness and the presence of numerous white cells, which are a response to the inflammation.

Treatment

The goals of treatment in rheumatoid arthritis are to provide relief from pain and to maintain or restore function of the arthritic joint. General treatment is similar to that for osteoarthritis, with the addition of some specific medications such as gold and oral corticosteroids. The same precautions given for injectable steroids apply to oral steroids, only more so. Hydroxychloroquine and penicillamine are two other disease-modifying antirheumatic medications, and immunosuppressive drugs such as azathioprine, cyclophosphamide, cyclosporine, and methotrexate are sometimes given for severe rheumatoid disease. Experimental therapies include intravenous immune gamma globulin (IgG) and interferon, biologic interventions that target specific immune reactions. Side effects from all these medications are many and can be severe. Their use must be closely monitored by a knowledgeable physician. A new drug, called Remicade, has been shown to potentiate the effects of methotrexate. One of the problems of Remicade is its expense; the first year's supply is expected to cost approximately $10,000.

A clinical trial delivering antiarthritis genes, which block the activity of metabolites implicated in the joint inflammation and destruction that characterizes rheumatoid arthritis, has been found both safe and effective in the treatment of the hands of patients with end-stage disease.

Synovectomy (removal of offending synovia) may sometimes provide relief. Total joint replacement can return a severely crippled rheumatoid patient to an active life by reducing pain and restoring movement.

Rheumatoid arthritis is a disease that is best treated by a team of health professionals that includes rheumatologists (arthritis specialists), physical and occupational therapists, social workers, and orthopaedic surgeons.

CASE REPORT—RHEUMATOID ARTHRITIS

Beatrice M. is a 32-year-old, red-haired woman with a fair complexion. Beatrice began to notice morning stiffness and pain on motion as well as tenderness in the small joints of her hands. Her fingers began to swell after several weeks, and then her feet also began to swell and ache. Involvement of the joints was always symmetric. Tender nodules appeared over the back of both her elbows. Beatrice began to lose her appetite and was fatigued enough to require a nap in the afternoon. She felt generally achy, stiff, and weak.

Beatrice's doctor took X-rays of her hands, which showed thinning of the bone next to her joints. Her blood tests showed that she was anemic, her sedimentation rate was elevated, and special blood examinations were positive for rheumatoid factors. A diagnosis of rheumatoid arthritis was made.

Beatrice was initially managed with high doses of aspirin, taken daily with food. She was placed on a program of physical therapy that included heat, massage, and gentle exercise. When her condition did not stabilize, she was started on gold therapy. She improved on this regimen, but the progress of the arthritis will be closely monitored and her disease may require more aggressive treatment if she does not continue to get better.

GOUT

Gout has affected such wise and famous men as Kubla Khan, Henry VIII, Goethe, Martin Luther, John Milton, Charlemagne, Oliver Cromwell, Galileo, Charles Darwin, Isaac Newton, William Pitt the Elder, and Theodore Roosevelt, to mention but a few. A goutlike disease of uric acid metabolism also affects the Dalmatian breed of pedigree dogs. Gout is no joke, despite cartoons of the gluttonous aristocrat, with his face contorted in pain and his swollen foot elevated on several pillows. This ancient disease, once called the rheumatism of the rich and now known to result from a metabolic flaw, is not caused by, but only aggravated by, overindulgence in food and drink.

Gouty arthritis is produced by an excess of uric acid in the body. Uric acid is the end product of the breakdown of certain foods. Although the patient with gout may present with pain in any joint, most typically the bunion joint of the large toe is painful. This involvement is called *podagra*, literally, "a foot attack:"

> Full soon the sad effect of this (port wine)
> His frame began to show
> For that old enemy the gout
> Had taken him in toe.
>
> *Thomas Hood, 1799–1845*

A blood test usually will show an elevated uric acid, and examination of fluid from an involved joint should reveal uric acid crystals. The accumulation of these crystals occasionally will cause what is known as a *gouty tophus* (L. "porous stone"), which sometimes has to be removed surgically.

The word *gout* originates from the Latin, *gutta*, meaning a drop, because the inflammation supposedly was due to the discharge—drop by drop—of harmful humors into the joints. We now know that gout is caused by either too much production or too little excretion of the metabolite uric acid. When this accumulates in or around the affected part (usually a joint), gouty attacks can be triggered by stress—gastronomic, physical, or emotional.

Gout plays no national favorites, even though the French claim they have the gouté for the taste, whereas the English have gout for the result. However, there is a strong gender predilection; more than 90 percent of gout sufferers are men, most of whom are highly achievement-oriented. This striking correlation between gout and prestige (it has been shown statistically that men with high IQs and increased blood uric acid levels are more likely to be leaders) has never been adequately explained.

Gout has been described in the bible: "And Esau in the thirty and ninth year of his reign was diseased in his feet, until his disease was exceedingly great: yet in his disease he sought not the Lord, but to the physician ..." (II Chronicles 16:12). In fact, Aaron's admonition to his sons that they not partake of wine else they die may refer to the association of severe attacks of gout with alcoholic intake.

The patient with gout should be under medical supervision. Advice given usually includes weight reduction and avoiding foods that are high in *purine*, a metabolic precursor of uric acid. These include organ foods, such as liver and kidney, as well as sardines.

A genetic factor may be involved in gout because some of the nearly 2 million Americans who suffer from the disease have specific enzyme deficiencies that lead to the condition.

People with gout are well advised to monitor and moderate their lifestyle, get plenty of rest and relaxation, and remain under medical supervision with a doctor who is familiar with the management of this disease. Gout was believed to be due not only to high living (a Spanish proverb says, "Gout is cured by walling up the mouth") but also to lechery. Benjamin Franklin, another notable gout sufferer, wrote, "Be temperate in wine, in eating, girls, and sloth, or the gout will seize you and plague you both" (*Poor Richard's Almanac*, 1734). Hippocrates, the father of medicine, states in his aphorisms, "Eunuchs do not take the gout, nor become bald.... A young man does not take the gout until he indulges in coition." Although overstated, there seems to be a measure of truth in these observations, because the process of gouty inflammation occurs mostly in the presence of male hormones.

The pain is almost unbearable and has been eloquently described by many great authors, including Jonathan Swift.

Dear Honest Ned is in the gout
Lies rackt with pain, and you without;

How patiently you hear him groan!
How glad the case is not your own!

State-of-the-art treatment consists of reasonable living habits, including proper diet and moderate exercise, because an episode of gout can be triggered by obesity, as well as by either too little or too much exercise with diminished fluid intake. To abort the acute episode, patients are given certain NSAIDs, cortisone, or colchicine, a drug known to the ancients as both a specific for easing the pain of gout and an assassin's poison that causes violent diarrhea and death. Further attacks can be prevented by drugs that either limit the production of uric acid or encourage its excretion. Some examples are probenecid and allopurinol.

With all the folklore, it sometimes is difficult to sort fact from fiction, but, venery and overeating apart, gout is very real to those who suffer it, and no joking matter!

CASE REPORT—GOUT

Alan G., a 46-year-old, overweight shoe salesman, presented with the sudden onset of redness, swelling, pain, and tenderness at the base of his left great toe. This attack of pain awakened him from a sound sleep in the middle of the night. That evening he had eaten a large dinner accompanied by copious amounts of red wine. Alan described the pain as a violent stretching and tearing alternating with tightening and pressure. He said that it was so severe that he couldn't even bear the weight of the bedsheets on the affected foot.

Alan was driven by a friend to the emergency room of his local hospital. There, radiographs demonstrated arthritis of the great toe with early cystic changes about the joint, and a blood test revealed a markedly elevated uric acid. A diagnosis of gout was made, and Alan was given colchicine. It took three tablets at hourly intervals before he began to sense relief of his pain. After the acute attack subsided, Alan was managed by his internist over the long term on a medication designed to lower his uric acid level. He was advised to reduce his weight, refrain from eating rich foods (particularly organ meats), restrict his alcohol intake, and discontinue smoking. He was told to get plenty of rest and try to avoid physical and emotional stress. His gout was easily managed on this regimen, and he has not had another acute attack.

OFFBEAT TREATMENT

Finally, a word about unusual treatments for arthritis. Henry VII's physician applied baked ox dung wrapped in cabbage leaves to his swollen joints, and even today many Americans suffering from arthritis are prime targets for questionable treatments and so-called arthritis cures. The Arthritis Foundation estimates that $950 million is wasted each year on worthless crack remedies. This amounts to $25 spent on unproved treatments for each $1 going toward bona fide research on rheumatic diseases. Such bogus cures take many forms, from copper bracelets to pyramid and aromatherapy. Not only are these treatments useless, but in addition to wasting your money some of them can be downright harmful. All of them delay effective therapy. If in doubt, contact your local Arthritis Foundation office and save yourself a lot of grief. You can reach the National Arthritis Foundation at 1-800-283-7800, or you can visit its World Wide Web site at http://www.arthritis.org, which provides a listing of local chapters as well as general information about arthritis.

QUESTIONS AND ANSWERS

Arthritis

Q: What are some of the unusual arthritic syndromes?

A: There are many. One is Reiter's syndrome, which is arthritis associated with urethritis (inflammation of the urethra), cervicitis (inflammation of the cervix), conjunctivitis (inflammation of the eyes), and mucocutaneous lesions (small, painless, superficial ulcers commonly seen in the mouth).

A German doctor, Hans Conrad Reiter, first described the syndrome in 1916. Because of his involvement in Nazi medical atrocities, the Spondylitis Association of America, a patient advocacy group representing patients with Reiter's syndrome, recently voted to rename this syndrome "reactive arthritis."

Christopher Columbus may have suffered from a form of arthritis accompanied by a low fever and painful eye inflammation during his third crossing (1498–1500) of the Atlantic. It was reported that in 1500, after a period of severe anxiety, all of his joints became swollen, and he had to be tied to the mast in bad weather to prevent his falling overboard. He died in 1506. The diagnosis of reactive arthritis has been suggested.

Another unusual type of arthritis is psoriatic arthritis, a rheumatoid-like arthritis associated with psoriasis of the skin or nails and a negative test for rheumatoid factor.

Yet another rare arthritic condition is Sjögren's syndrome. This is a chronic systemic inflammatory disorder of unknown etiology. It is characterized by dryness of the eyes, mouth, and other mucous membranes, and often is associated with rheumatic disorders showing certain autoimmune features.

Q: Is rheumatic fever a form of arthritis?

A: No. Rheumatic fever is an acute inflammatory complication of group A streptococcal infections. It is characterized mainly by arthritis, chorea (involuntary rapid, highly complex, jerky movements), or carditis (inflammation of the heart), appearing alone or in combination. Residual heart disease is a possible sequela of the carditis. Skin lesions may be found.

Q: What is hemorrhagic joint disease?

A: Hemorrhagic joint disease is found in hemophiliacs. Minor trauma can cause bleeding into a joint with subsequent damage because the blood does not clot. Arthritic changes can occur with repeated episodes.

Q: Can infections cause arthritis?

A: By all means. Both bacterial joint infections and tuberculosis can lead to joint damage and subsequent arthritis. This is also true of fungus infections, gonorrhea, and even syphilis.

Q: What is pseudogout?

A: Pseudogout is a joint disease with protean (many) manifestations. These may include intermittent episodes of acute arthritis as well as a degenerative arthropathy (joint pathology) that is often severe but can be asymptomatic (without symptoms). There is X-ray evidence of calcification of the articular cartilage (chondrocalcinosis) in characteristic sites. This is due to the deposition of a mineral crystal called calcium pyrophosphate dihydrate. The cause is not known.

Q: Are there distinctive diseases that include arthritis as a finding?

A: Lyme disease (tick-borne), *Salmonella* food poisoning, scleroderma, and lupus are a few of the many diseases that can involve the joints and include arthritis as a symptom or finding. In the case of *Salmonella* food poisoning, the immune system, whose job is to destroy infectious agents, does this by attacking a protein in the *Salmonella* organism., But that protein resembles one found in normal cells, so a confused immune system attacks that too, causing the painful joint inflammation of arthritis.

Q: Can the temporomandibular (jaw) joint be involved with arthritis?

A: Most forms of arthritis can involve the temporomandibular joint, including osteo-, infectious, traumatic, and rheumatoid arthritis. Any of these conditions can cause ankylosis (fusion) of this joint. The temporomandibular joint also can suffer congenital and developmental anomalies. More common is a myofascial pain and/or dysfunction syndrome of the joint. This condition is psychophysiologic, usually resulting from tension-relieving, jaw-clenching, or tooth-grinding habits.

Q: What is pigmented villonodular synovitis?

A: Pigmented villonodular synovitis is a condition in which the synovial tissue of joints, bursae, and tendon sheaths becomes thickened and covered with long, tangled, rubbery nodules. It typically is a disease of adults, and although its etiology is unclear, an inflammation of unknown origin is the most commonly accepted cause. The knee is the customary site of involvement. Pressure indentation and sometimes actual destruction of bone can occur late in the disease. The predominant symptom is a chronic swelling of the joint associated with mild aching. Bleeding into the joint may occur. The condition is benign, and the treatment is complete synovectomy (removal of the synovia). If all involved synovia has been removed, the joint is cured and a new, healthy synovia will grow back in short order.

I repeatedly mentioned exercise in this chapter. Before we consider its use in the treatment of specific joints, I want you to gain some understanding of its importance and the rudiments of its practice. Read on.

3

Exercise

"Health is the vital principle of bliss,
And exercise, of health."
James Thomson (1700–1748)
The Castle of Indolence
Canto I, Stanza 55

The exercise prescription is so important to the health of your joints that it deserves a chapter all to itself. Other sections of this book inform you about specific exercises for the joint under consideration. This chapter sketches the broad picture of exercise and its importance in maintaining health.

The imperative to move is inborn in all children. Even though a child's motor nerves are not fully developed until the age of five years and sometimes even later, much earlier physical stimulation through exercise can help develop motor skills such as balance and coordination. Motor activity can be facilitated and patterns of movement stimulated in newborns and infants. This assists them in developing self-awareness through movement. The ability to sit and later stand and walk is accelerated through muscle strengthening. Making the infant aware of the role of the feet in supporting his or her body assists him or her in standing, and walking is encouraged by balancing exercises. One such program is the system of graduated exercise that begins with relaxation and then incorporates gymnastics in preparation for sitting, as well as exercise play to prepare for standing. This excellent method, which uses play to prepare for independent movement, was developed by Dr. Janine Lévy (*The Baby Exercise Book*, Pantheon Books, 1973).

AGING

John Dryden (1631–1700) wrote, "The wise for cure on exercise depend...." How true. It has been said that if exercise were available in a pill, it would be prescribed for almost every patient and every medical condition. Activity of muscles is necessary for protein synthesis and simply keeping up with the normal muscular loss related to aging (called sarcopenia: Gr. flesh-poverty) requires the exercise prescription. At complete bedrest, strength is lost at approximately 3 to 5 percent each day. After age 30, your total number of muscle fibers begins to decline, reducing muscle strength by up to 30 percent when you reach the age of 60. Between the ages of 30 and 80 years, the strength of the leg, arm, and back muscles can decrease as much as 60 percent, reflecting a progressive decrement of muscle with as much as 10 to 15 percent loss per decade after age 50. New research shows that we not only lose muscle mass as we age but also a larger percentage of "fast-twitch" muscle fibers associated with reaction time and quickness. A senior citizen with fewer "fast-twitch" fibers has trouble avoiding falls. But proper exercise, particularly weight training, can maintain "fast-twitch" fibers and even bring them back. It is known that neuromuscular changes and decreased levels of body hormones are partly responsible for this deterioration. However, the major contributor is reduced exercise, particularly workouts using weights or exercising against resistance. Endurance also decreases, leading to fatigue. Animal studies have found that the ability of muscles to provide sustained power diminishes by 50 percent with age. This appears to be due to a loss of *mitochondria* (the energy factories of the cell), which in turn results in a decline in enzyme-linked oxidative capacity (the ability to utilize oxygen to provide energy). Older muscles are more easily injured and take longer to recover. Protracted healing lengthens the period of immobility due to pain. These weakened muscles are vulnerable to injury, and a vicious cycle of weakness-injury-pain-weakness occurs. Muscles lose strength rapidly with prolonged rest, and normal power may never return.

Muscular vigor is reduced as aerobic capacity decreases with age. This physiologic decline begins at about age 30. From then on, the ability of the heart to pump declines by approximately 1 percent per year. Blood vessels are nearly 30 percent narrower by middle age, decreasing blood flow in the limbs by 30 to 60 percent by age 60. After age 30, the force of gravity begins to overpower weakening muscles in the stomach and back. This leads to gradual compression of the intervertebral discs, resulting in a decrease in height. In addition, the tensile strength of ligaments is diminished, adding to injury propensity in the elderly.

The good news is that this trend can be reversed through exercise! Numerous studies have shown that a graded, well-supervised exercise program, including both strength training and aerobic drill, can lead to significant functional improvement in such parameters as gait velocity, stair-climbing, and spontaneous physical activity in the middle-aged, and even in individuals over 70 years of age.

Hypertension, congestive heart failure, coronary artery disease, type II diabetes, osteoporosis, osteoarthritis, and cognitive disorders such as Alzheimer's disease, as well as ischemic (reduced blood supply) strokes, are more prevalent as people age. In addition to delaying the onset of many of these conditions, regular exercise can improve function and delay infirmity and disability in those who have them. Regular exercise may work synergistically with medication to combat the effects of some chronic diseases. According to studies at Johns Hopkins University, each stair you climb adds four seconds to your life.

Exercise also helps keep the body trim. Our primary fuel is fat, one pound providing 3,500 calories. It is almost impossible to burn that off at "one fell swoop" unless you run a marathon. This is because the muscles use sugar for energy before they tap into your stores of fat. Actually, your body is extremely efficient in converting food into fuel. For example, riding a bicycle at 10 mph for one hour requires only three ounces of carbohydrate. This is the energy equivalent to about 1.4 ounces of gasoline. If we used gasoline instead of food, we could ride more than 900 miles on a single gallon! Sugar, utilized more easily, is stored in the muscles and therefore recruited first. But there isn't very much sugar immediately available, so it quickly runs out. In contrast, fat is stored at a distance from the muscles and is harder to access when you first start to exercise. However, fat is almost inexhaustible. Ultimately, both sugar and fat provide the energy used to make *ATP* (adenosine triphosphate—the molecule providing energy for muscles), and the energy from ATP is then used to contract muscles. The various chemical energy systems of muscle are covered in detail in my book *All About Muscle* (Demos, 2000).

LOSING FAT

Exercise helps you lose fat because it increases the body's use of calories. One hour of vigorous activity can use up to 600 calories, the equivalent of a hamburger and a milkshake. A 150-pound individual will burn up to 13.2 calories by running fast for one minute, 8.1 calories by swimming, and 6.35 calories by bicycling, and 6.6 calories are utilized each minute by aerobic exercise. Walking metabolizes only 3.8 calories in the same time. Most people walk 3,000 to 4,000 steps a day. If you can increase this to 10,000 steps a day, you can burn an extra 1,500 calories a week. Using a pedometer will keep you aware of your extra steps during the day. You begin to realize that taking the stairs instead of an elevator or walking instead of driving the three blocks to the grocery store really does make a difference. A 150-pound person chopping with an axe at a fast pace for one hour will use up 1,212 calories, performing judo 798, cross-country skiing 486, playing basketball 564, golfing 348, and playing billiards 174 calories. At the same time, you are moving your joints; stretching muscle, tendon, and ligaments; increasing circulation to the joints utilized in the exercise; and increasing strength, endurance, and agility.

Exercise builds lean body mass as it burns excess fatty tissue. The percentage of body fat is kept at an appropriate level. What confuses people on an exercise program at first is they may not lose as many pounds as they hope to lose because they have lost fat but gained muscle. Then they realize "Hey, my hips and waist are slimmer!" Exercise increases thirst but can decrease appetite. It helps to remember that the feeling of being hungry can sometimes be satiated by drinking, particularly a warm fluid such as weak tea. Finally, exercise increases the body's metabolic rate (the rate at which the bodily processes work) for up to six hours, so that you continue to burn up more calories after as well as during your exercise. Exercise can cause micro-tears in muscle fibers. After exercising, the body repairs this 'damage," building the muscles even stronger. As muscle is built, more calories are required to nourish it. The end result is that the body will burn more calories from fat.

A German proverb has it that "he who goes for a walk lengthens the way to his grave."

Exercise indeed improves every organ in the body.

- ❏ The liver responds by producing glycogen more efficiently.
- ❏ Insulin and glucose are better regulated by the pancreas.
- ❏ More oxygen is delivered by the lungs, and the heart pumps more strongly.
- ❏ The circulatory system builds more capillaries.
- ❏ The level of bad cholesterol in the blood drops while the level of good cholesterol increases.
- ❏ Bones respond by becoming denser.
- ❏ The mitochondria that produce ATP enlarge.
- ❏ The muscles learn to burn more and more fat

Here are some myths about exercise that should be dispelled:

1. *If a little exercise is good, more is better.*

Those over 60 years of age need exercise to only 70 percent of their capacity to derive maximum benefits. Overexercising is not practical and can be dangerous.

2. *Exercise leaves you in pain and fatigued.*

An unsupervised exercise binge can, of course, exhaust you and make your muscles sore. Regular exercise that is well scheduled relaxes you and increases energy.

3. *Exercise can cause a heart attack.*

After years of sedentary living, a sudden burst of intense exercise can put strain on your heart. However, regular exercise reasonably performed develops a healthier heart and can ward off a heart attack.

4. *Hard work can make you age.*

Working so hard that you can just about drag yourself to bed can wear anyone out, but a regular exercise program produces changes in the body that slow the aging process.

5. *For exercise to be effective, you have to work out many hours each day.*

Studies have shown that exercise two to threetimes a week for a minimum of 20 to 30 minutes is all that is necessary to maintain fitness.

A complete exercise program includes:

❏ Endurance exercises that are aerobic in nature. These exercises condition your cardiovascular system and lungs and help you relax. They may include a walking or jogging regimen. Seventy percent of Americans own running shoes but don't run. Don't be one of them!
❏ Strengthening exercises are necessary for posture and balance. Selected calisthenics are programmed. Weight training is essential.
❏ Range of motion exercises, including stretching, are designed to improve joint mobility.

SCHEDULING

Early in the morning or late in the afternoon usually is the best time to exercise. Exercising at midday may be bad in the summer because of the heat. Muscle strength, aerobic capacity, and flexibility are all at their peak between 3 P.M. and 4 P.M. A minimum of two to three and a maximum of five workouts each week is adequate. These can be performed anywhere. Your bedroom is a good place for stretching exercises. Carpeting may provide enough padding, or you can purchase an exercise mat. Walking and jogging should be done in the most pleasant surroundings possible. Proper running shoes must be worn, and it is best to run on springy turf or cinder if at all possible. Exercise is possible year-round if you wear appropriate clothing. A workout can be particularly invigorating in moderately cold weather. Apparel should be loose and layered for outdoor exercise so that the outer layer can be peeled off as you warm up and sweat. You must sweat if you are to benefit from exercising.

It is important to check with your physician before beginning any exercise program. If you make any significant changes in your level of physical activity, you should again check with your doctor. Remember to take it slow in the beginning and know your limit. This means exercising at a rate within your capacity.

You must warm up before you work out in order to increase blood flow to your muscles. Gradually starting up in this manner helps prevent injury because soft tissues are most easily damaged when they are cold. You should cool down after the workout because your circulation needs to readjust. Five minutes of walking after a jog usually will suffice.

Don't shower immediately after exercising because a hot shower can open up the circulation just like vigorous activity does. Delay your post-workout shower for at least 5 to 10 minutes, and even then you should make the shower warm, not excessively hot. If you exercise with others, don't compete, and never overexert yourself. Overexercising stimulates adrenaline, which decreases the efficiency of the heart. Don't exercise if you are sick, as exercise challenges your body to reach its full potential and you need all your strength to heal your illness. If you have even a slight cold, your physiology has enough to do without overloading it with exercise. Eat lightly before exercising, but don't skip meals because your body requires nutrition to fuel its activity.

SOME EXERCISE POINTERS

- ❏ Don't bounce during stretching.
- ❏ Avoid vigorous overarching of the back, and don't exercise with your knees locked.
- ❏ All muscles act in sets, and exercise should be aimed at balancing the use of these muscle pairs.
- ❏ Stretching and strengthening muscles is the object of proper exercise.
- ❏ Pay attention while you are exercising. Develop muscle awareness. Let your body guide you. Remember that movement is natural and has a healing quality. Nowadays patients are encouraged to move about within 24 hours after an operation.
- ❏ During stretching, stretch just a bit beyond the point of fatigue.
- ❏ Don't exercise too fast or you will overload your joints.
- ❏ Avoid deep knee bends or stretch situps or pushups.

THE EXERCISE PRESCRIPTION

It is never too early and seldom too late to begin an exercise program that will prevent or even reverse age-related problems. Exercise can maintain proper joint nutrition and mobility in osteoarthritis. The risk of cardiopulmonary illness is reduced with aerobic exercise. General fitness can be maintained by following a proper exercise prescription.

A long-term goal of 30 minutes of brisk walking or other aerobic exercise at least three times a week is ideal. Regular walking with a partner keeps you both motivated. If you can hold a normal conversation without losing your breath while you are walking, your pace is just about right. If walking is too strenuous, you can exercise from a chair in the beginning. Moving rhythmically while seated provides aerobic exercise. Getting up from a chair a number of times works the leg muscles and has a built-in safety factor. If you tend to fall backward, the chair will stop you. Seniors can improve their balance and soon will be walking better. A step aerobic platform can provide a stable base to put next to the kitchen counter. This can be used as a step for quadriceps and hamstring strengthening.

If you live in a high-rise elevator building, you need not always take the elevator. Try walking up one flight and down two flights, and then take the elevator. When the weather is bad, you can walk the apartment house corridors back and forth, starting with your floor, then take the stairs down a flight, and walk back and forth again. Walk down another flight of stairs, and so forth.

Dancing is another enjoyable exercise that can engage you to take your exercise prescription. It has excellent aerobic potential and a low risk of injury as well as the added benefit of providing the social interaction that is crucial for older adults.

An adult who finds exercise boring will abandon it just as quickly as a youngster will. The stationary cycle is a mainstay for those who have poor vision and/or an unsteady gait. Cycling can be made more interesting by watching television or playing a favorite recording while exercising. Any number of special adaptations make enjoyable exercise available for the older person. Low-intensity exercise (e.g., fewer repetitions), low-impact exercise (e.g., cycling or exercise while sitting), and modified equipment (smaller weights, special shoes, loose clothing) will all help. Moving rhythmically while seated provides aerobic exercise. "Chair dancing" is a gentle but active alternative exercise program. For information, contact Chair Dancing, Dept. P, 2658 Del Mar Heights Road, Del Mar, CA 92014; phone 800/551-4386.

If you're in good shape, walking faster or walking uphill can add a bit of aerobic intensity to your walk. Simply swinging your arms while walking increases your heart rate and the number of calories burned. In fact, just vigorously swinging the arms provides good aerobic exercise for cardiovascular conditioning. Symphonic orchestra conductors are notably long-lived because they "jarm" in this fashion. You can do the same thing with a recording of your favorite fast-moving classical record. Try it!

Using weighted gloves, wrist weights, and hand weights (but not heavier than three pounds) can raise your heart rate by 5 to 15 beats per minute and boost caloric expenditure 15 percent as long as you swing your arms. Just carrying the weights does nothing. Be advised that weights heavier than three pounds can strain your neck, shoulders, and arms. Gripping hand weights can elevate your blood pressure. Don't use ankle weights or weighted vests because these can cause pain or injury to the lower extremities. A power belt can be worn around the waist. This has resistive cords with handles to pull as you walk. The use of the power belt increases upper body strength, heart rate, and caloric expenditure by more than 50 percent, which makes it too intense for all but very serious, younger fitness walkers. Walking poles are like ski poles with rubber tips. They weigh less than a pound each. They elevate the heart rate by 10 to 20 beats per minute and increase the number of calories burned by up to 25 percent. The poles also support your weight and reduce pressure on the feet by 25 percent. They are ideal for overweight people or those with lower extremity problems. The equipment mentioned here can be purchased through any large sporting goods store.

Resistance exercise should be started with a very light load. Lifting exercises should be executed rapidly because this will increase your ability to perform the explosive movements necessary to rise from a chair or catch your balance. On the other hand, if your goal is to increase strength, you should use lighter weights and lift at about one-third the normal speed ("super-slow"). This forces you to fully contract the muscles you're working through their full range of motion. It is reasonable to allow

6 to 8 weeks before you notice any change. If you expect immediate improvement, you will become discouraged and discontinue your exercise regimen.

A complete program of strengthening can be provided with a modest investment in very simple equipment, such as plastic-coated dumbbells and rubber tubing and elastic bands, or by joining a health club. A stationary exercise bicycle, stepmaster, or cross-country Nordic ski machine can provide adequate resistance as well as endurance training. A treadmill can substitute for a vigorous walk. Walking in waist-high water in a swimming pool will provide effective resistance, and water aerobics are an excellent form of exercise, particularly for seniors.

BALANCE EXERCISES

Balance exercises as simple as alternately standing on each foot or the use of a wobble board stimulate *proprioceptive feedback* (tactile and position sense) through mechanoreceptors arrayed about your joints. Exercising on a moving bicycle is better than the same amount of pedaling on a stationary bike because you are practicing the ability to balance. Research studies have shown that nursing home residents enrolled in a program of balancing exercises including Tai-chi (slow Oriental drill) movement suffered far fewer falls with subsequent broken bones than those who did not participate.

We lose "functional reserve" as we grow older, and every year about 30 percent of people over age 65 and 50 percent of those over age 80 fall. Almost 10 percent of those who fall are seriously hurt. Fractures among women 65 years and older increased 40 percent between 1988 and 1996. Each year more adults over age 65 die from fall-related injuries than from any other cause. Some 4,000 such deaths occurred in 1997. One in three older adults requires hospitalization for a fall each year. A broken hip is the most common and most serious injury. Half of those who break a hip fail to regain their former level of mobility and independence, moving in with relatives or ending up in a nursing home.

However, the balance reflex mechanism can always be improved. Therapies and preventive measures are available for anyone with balance problems. Balance exercise can be as easy as standing at a sink holding onto the sides and rising to your tiptoes, and then slowly lowering yourself. You can practice getting out of a chair four to five times without using your hands or making it a goal to walk a little further each day. The American Physical Therapy Association is a good resource for information to help seniors avoid falls and get answers to questions about balance and exercise. They can be contacted by writing to the American Physical Therapy Association, 1111 North Fairfax Street, Alexandria, VA 22314; 703/684-2982; fax 703/684-7343.

Few good reasons but many excuses are offered by seniors who don't want to exercise. I list some of the most frequently offered here, with an appropriate response. These have been adopted from a multisite field test of the acceptability of physical activity, counseling, and primary care: Project PACE. This was conducted by Long BJ, Calfas KJ, Wooten W et al. It was published in the *American Journal of Preventive Medicine*, Volume 12, No. 2, 1996, and adapted in an article, "Overcoming exercise barriers in older adults," by Drs. Jay Dunlap and Harry C. Barry, published in *The Physician and Sports Medicine*, Volume 27, No. 11, October 15, 1999.

EXCUSE	RESPONSE
"Exercise is hard."	You can start with ordinary walking or an exercise that is not work for most people. See where it might lead.
"I don't have the time."	That may be true, but you will never know for sure unless you try to make the time.
"I'm usually too tired for exercise."	You should tell yourself, "this activity will give me more energy." See if it doesn't happen.
"I hate to fail, so I hesitate to start."	Physical activity is not a test. You won't fail if you choose an activity you like and start slowly. Setting reasonable, realistic goals reduces the chance of failure.

continued on next page

EXCUSE	RESPONSE
"I don't have anyone to work out with."	Maybe you have not asked enough people. A neighbor or coworker may be a willing partner, or you could choose an activity that you enjoy doing alone. Better yet, join a gym or health club. This is an ideal way to socialize while keeping fit.
"I don't have a convenient place to exercise."	Pick an activity that you can do at a convenient place. Walk around your neighborhood or a nearby mall, or do exercise with a TV show or videotape.
"I am afraid of being injured."	Walking is a very safe and excellent exercise. Wear comfortable shoes, and choose a safe, well-lighted area. You might also want to take "aquacise" classes at a "Y" or health club, a safe and enjoyable way to initiate an exercise program
"The weather is too bad."	You can do many activities in your own home or at a shopping mall in any kind of weather.
"Exercise is boring."	There are ways to make exercise more fun. These include exercising with a companion, varying the exercise with the season, setting a non–exercise-related goal such as getting an errand or two done in the course of it or giving yourself a periodic reward.
"I am too fat."	You can benefit regardless of your weight. Pick an activity that you are comfortable doing, such as walking.
"I am just too old."	It is never too late to start. People of any age can benefit from exercise.

STRETCHING

You must stretch to limber up before you excercuse. Stretching helps to avoid injury by maintaining flexibility. With flexible joints it is easier to avoid injury that may necessitate surgery or other medical treatment. One study of more than 100 people complaining of foot pain concluded that many who were advised to have corrective surgical procedures could avoid such operations if they regularly stretched their Achilles (heel) tendons. Much low back pain can be prevented or eliminated by properly stretching the muscles of the lower back and the hamstring muscles on the back of the thighs (Chart 3-1).

STRETCHING EXERCISES

Here are some good stretching exercises that can be used as a general warmup for any sports activity, such as running, swimming, tennis, and so forth. They are also useful for cooling down after the activity.

1. Lie comfortably on your back with your knees bent. Take a deep breath and, exhaling, slide your right foot forward and back. Repeat with the left foot. Clench your fists tightly, then relax.

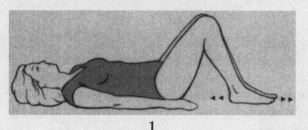

1

2. Lying on your back with the knees bent, breathe in and out deeply and slowly. Pull your shoulders up with every inhalation. Relax as you exhale.

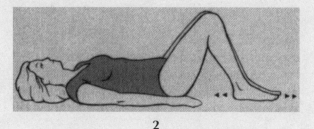

2

3. In the same position, turn your head as far to the right as possible. Return to the normal position and relax. Repeat the exercise turning your head to the left.

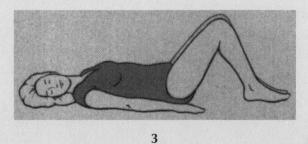

3

4. Lie on your back with your knees bent and pull both knees up to your chest. Lower them slowly to the floor.

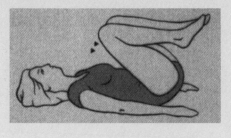

4

5. While kneeling with the wight resting on your hands and knees, arch your back, at the same time dropping your head.

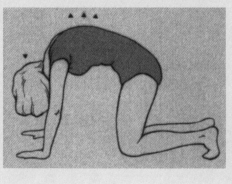

5

6. Still in the kneeling position, place your weight on your hands and knees. Gradually slide your arms forward until your forearms are resting on the floor. Move slowly back to the original position.

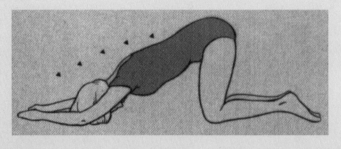

6

7. Lying on your back with your knees bent, place your hands on your abdomen and raise your head, your neck, and finally your shoulders from the floor. Return slowly to the starting position and repeat.

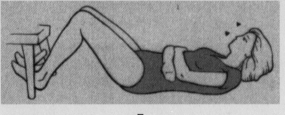

7

8. Lying on your back with your knees bent, first bring your left knee to your chest, then extend the left leg with toes pointed toward the ceiling. Keeping your left knee straight, lower the leg to the floor, then bring it back up to the flexed position. Repeat these movements with the opposite leg.

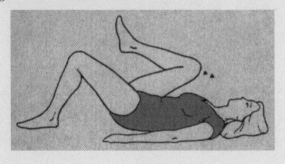

8

9. Still lying on your back with your knees bent, slide your left leg forward. With the knee locked, perform a straight leg lift, raising the leg as high as possible. Lower the leg slowly to the floor, slide it to the flexed position, and repeat with the opposite leg.

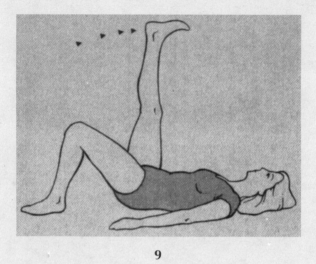

9

10. Standing with the heels together and the hands behind the back, bend slowly forward from the hips, moving down as far as you can.

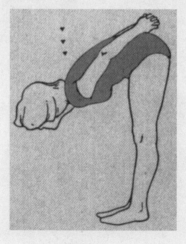

10

11. Stand an arm's length from a wall with both feet together, place your hands flat on the wall and keep your hips and knees straight. Using your hands and forearms for support, try to place your chest on the wall. You will feel a stretch in your heel cords. Straighten your arms and push your body back to the original position.

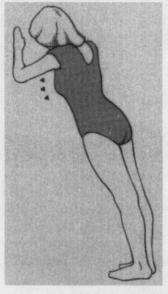

11

12. Standing with your heels together, take a deep breath. While you let it out slowly, bend forward from the waist, dropping your head, shoulders, and finally your hips. Do not force this exercise. You should feel some stretch in your back and the back of your legs. Relax and straighten up.

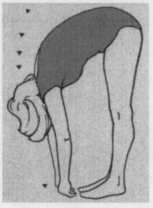

12

When should you stretch? If possible, both before and after exercising. Stretching should not hurt, although you should feel a gentle pull. The admonition "no pain, no gain" should be buried. Don't have someone else passively force the stretch beyond your pain threshold. Don't bounce when you stretch. Each stretch should be held for 30 seconds. Stretching beyond 30 seconds adds no benefit. Of course, you should slowly work up to the 30 seconds if you can't reach that level the first time you stretch. Your local "Y" or health club may offer stretch classes.

POSITION SENSE

Osteoarthritis of the knee currently affects some 3 million Americans, mostly those over age 60. This condition responds to exercise. It has long been thought that people with osteoarthritis of the knee have a weak quadriceps (upper leg) muscle as a result of the disease. The theory was that the pain caused by the arthritis prevented people from moving about and the muscle wasted because it wasn't used. However, it now appears that weak thigh muscles are a *cause* rather than a result of osteoarthritis of the knee. People with strong quadriceps muscles are able to control how hard they impact with the ground when they walk, thereby reducing stress on the knees. Those with weak quadriceps lack control and tend to impact harder when they walk or run. Unnecessary stress is placed on the knee, leading to a breakdown of the cartilage that cushions the joint. Loss of joint alignment occurs, and *proprioception* (joint position sense) is decreased, initiating a vicious cycle of further damage. In carefully controlled studies, a program of quadriceps-strengthening exercise resulted in significant improvement in patients with osteoarthritis of the knee (Chart 3-2). The use of a light elastic or neoprene knee sleeve can also be beneficial in providing proprioceptive input.

SOME EXERCISE AIDS

Exercise videos are helpful in initiating and following an exercise program. Many are currently available. I suggest that you borrow some from your local library and see which suits your particular time and need. The Jane Fonda video is very popular

---

QUADRICEPS STRENGTHENING KNEE MUSCLE EXERCISES

1. Lie on your back on a firm, flat surface, keeping your knee perfectly straight and stiff (180 degrees). Lift the leg as high as possible. Slowly return the leg to the resting position. Relax momentarily.

During this exercise, tension should be felt in the muscles of the front of the thigh. Do as many straight leg lifts as possible the first day. Gradually increase the number you can perform by adding one repetition each succeeding day to a maximum of fifty lifts. Continue with fifty lifts daily. Proceed slowly; you may feel fatigued but should not experience pain.

2. Comfortably seated with a shoe on, hook the foot of the involved knee under a desk, sofa, chair, or other piece of furniture too heavy to lift. Keeping the knee perfectly straight and stiff, attempt to lift the furniture, exerting a maximal effort and slowly counting to six. Relax. During the exercise, tension should be felt in the muscles of the front of the thigh. Next, bend the knee approximately 30 degrees, and repeat the exercise. Finally, bend the knee approximately 60 degrees, and repeat again.

These are isometric exercises. The knee should not move during the six-second maximal contracture. Each exercise is to be performed only once during an exercise period. Repeat these isometric exercises three times a day.

for aerobic exercise, and the Karen Voight fitness videos, especially the ones on stretching, have garnered positive reviews from exercise scientists.

Two- to four-pound plastic-covered dumbbells are excellent for exercising the forearms and shoulders. At the same time we need to overload our muscles by repetitively lifting at least 60 percent of the maximum amount we can lift at one time. If muscle growth is your main goal, three sets of 8 to 10 repetitions is the optimal routine. A modified pushup (with the knees on the floor) can be quite effective in building strength in the shoulders. The legs have the largest muscles in the body (60 percent of our muscle mass), and they should be exercised for stamina and to help burn more calories. Squats are intended to strengthen the quadriceps muscles. When squatting, you should bend no more than 90 degrees. It can help to keep your back against the wall when you start these squats. In fact, a simple way to measure muscle strength is to stand with your knees slightly bent against a door or a wall that has a slick surface. Lower your body as far as you can with the back supported by the wall (but do not flex the knees beyond 90 degrees) and then rise again. This "sit-and-rise-test" gives a rough indication of strength and provides a baseline for measuring strength training progress. Don't forget, deep knee bends are forbidden!

Believe it or not, sex is an efficient calorie-burner. A 125-pound woman can burn up to 4.5 calories per minute during intercourse. Sex also enhances muscle tone, and it's a great cardiovascular workout. During sex, heart rate can reach 125 beats per minute. Obviously, it can be too stressful if it's illicit or unsafe.

An alert person can find many opportunities to exercise during his or her daily routine. Here are some suggestions.

❑ Take every opportunity to walk. Without even trying, the average person will walk 75,000 miles in his or her lifetime, or three times around the world! So you've got a good start.

❑ Now continue your round-the-world marathon by walking whenever you can. The walking speed of the average American woman is 256 feet per minute (of the average man 245 feet per minute). See if you can step this up a bit.

❏ Walk up and down stairs instead of taking elevators. It has been estimated that each stair you climb adds four seconds to your life.

❏ Lift and carry reasonable loads rather than using wheelbarrows or carts (but always remember proper technique, lifting from the knees and not from the back).

❏ Tighten your abdomen. Try to bring your belly button to your backbone, and hold it very tight for a slow count of six when you are seated in your car waiting for the stoplight to change. In addition to toning your abs, this will take an inch or two off your waistline.

❏ Perform simple isometric exercises at your desk each day. This involves contracting muscle without moving joints, as contrasted with isotonic contraction, in which joints are moved. These exercises can include pressing your hands together, pulling your hands apart, pressing your knees together, pushing your knees apart against the resistance provided by your hands, lifting yourself by your hands in a firm chair, pushing away from your desk, bending your head to each side against resistance provided from an outstretched palm, and so forth. Each of these isometric positions should be held for a slow count of six. You will have to use 75 percent of your strength before you get any benefit, so try to exert a maximal contraction when exercising isometrically like this.

A plan for workplace stretching exercises is described in "Stretching at your Computer or Desk," by Bob Anderson, which is available at bookstores or from Stretching, Inc., Box 767, Dept. P, Palmer Lake, Colorado 80133-0767 (1/800/333-1307), www.stretching.com on the web.

AEROBIC EXERCISE

An anonymous wag once said, "I have two doctors—my left leg and my right." Aerobic exercise, or exercise that calls upon your cardiovascular system (heart, lungs, and blood vessels) while using oxygen, has an effect on the entire body. It improves your heart, lungs, liver, and bones. It increases endurance and enhances general health. In order to be effective, aerobic exercise must use the muscles of the legs, make your heart beat faster, and induce deep breathing. It is called *aerobic* because it uses lots of oxygen. Uninterrupted exercise for about 15 minutes is ideal, but you can gain aerobic benefits by simply running in place as fast as you can for one to three minutes. This works your legs, makes you breathe deeply, and increases your heart rate. You always continue to metabolize fat after exercise, but you only metabolize fat directly *while* exercising if the exercise is aerobic. This becomes very important when we realize that the chances that an American adult is obese are 1 in 4.

The heart is a highly specialized muscle. It contracts like any other muscle, metabolizes fat as well, and depends on glycogen (sugar) for energy. The body has a mechanism that preferentially directs its metabolism to replenish glycogen for the heart before other muscles are served. Even though the blood may be loaded with glucose (glycogen precursor), other muscles do not get any until the needs of the heart are satisfied. If any sugar is left over, the glycogen storehouse in the liver begins to fill. No one knows exactly how this mechanism works. It is another example of the mystery and miracle of the human body.

ACTIVE REST

Recovery after injury is *not* hastened by rest. This is because injured joints are particularly vulnerable to long absence from movement. Without exercise, soft tissue about a joint tightens, causing pain when motion is attempted. Because of this, a program of "active rest" has been proposed by sports medicine professionals. This seeks a balance between the activity that has caused the injury and the underuse that is likely to worsen it. Active rest for a running injury of the knee might be swimming or walking. Active rest for a strained back involves special exercise and returning to work (assuming that you're not a professional furniture mover) as soon as possible. Varying your exercise program provides the brief periods of rest that muscles need.

INCREASING STRENGTH

Recent studies have shown that a two-month strengthening program in men and women aged 60 to 96 increased the strength of the 60- and 70-year-olds by 200 percent and the size of their muscles by 15 percent. Those in their nineties experienced a 180 percent gain in strength while their muscles grew by 12 percent. In addition, their bones became denser and their joints more mobile.

Weak muscles are poorly supplied with oxygen. They tire easily when you attempt to work them, and they ache and want to rest. Muscular exhaustion occurs because muscle fibers run out of the oxygen needed to extract energy from sugar and fat. Working a muscle builds circulation so that more oxygen is delivered to the muscle factory. Strength and endurance increase, and limbs that are stronger allow you to avoid accidents—from dropping things to stumbling, spraining your joints, and breaking your bones.

A muscle's ability to use oxygen increases with an increase in temperature. That is why warming up is important before exercise. Also, warm muscles are less susceptible to being injured because they are more elastic. Higher temperatures improve the function of nerves. As the capillaries in the muscle dilate with warming, more blood carrying more oxygen is brought to the muscles for the removal of waste products such as carbon dioxide and lactic acid. The heart also benefits from warming up. Cardiac irregularities on an electrocardiogram are often decreased by warming up. Finally, fat is burned more efficiently in muscles that have been warmed up.

WOMEN AND EXERCISE

Strength training does not cause women to become muscle-bound. Instead, such training reduces body fat. Lean body mass weighs more than fat, so a slight increase in weight may occur with exercise. Strength training does not produce any significant increase in lower body girth and only a slight increase in the size of the upper extremities.

Women should be encouraged to train at high intensity because light training is often below what is necessary for physiologic adaptation in body tissues. Finally, women can use the same training methods as men because they are no more likely to be injured during strength training. Sport-specific exercise should take into consideration the biomechanics of the sport for which a female athlete is training.

Strength training benefits for women include a higher metabolic rate, increased functional strength for daily activity and athletic participation, decreased body fat, increased lean body muscle mass, stronger connective tissues (ligaments and tendons), increased bone modeling and strength with a subsequent reduction in the risk of osteoporosis (weakness of bone), and enhanced confidence and self-esteem. The Women's Sports Foundation is a nonprofit national organization established by Billie Jean King and Donna de Varona in 1974 to increase opportunities for females in sport and fitness. Members include such world-class athletes as Chris Evert, Bonnie Blair, Jackie Joyner-Kersee, Rebecca Lobo, and Camille Duvall, but anyone can join. Through its conferences, newsletter (*Sports Talk*), and materials, girls and women can learn how to balance sports and life and stay motivated. The foundation also offers annual cash awards for travel and training to female athletes of all ages and ability. To learn more, write: The Women's Sports Foundation, Eisenhower Park, East Meadow, NY 11554, or visit www.womenssportfoundation. org on the web.

NATURAL EXERCISE

Exercising out of doors provides benefits that exercising on a machine does not. It's more fun and calls upon the body to balance, adding a cross-training effect. If you run on a trail rather than on a treadmill, you have to adjust to irregularities in the running surface, and even sometimes run uphill, which gives a wind-sprint effect. It is better to walk or to jog with occasional short bursts of effort in the middle. These spurts of intensity tend to burn fat more efficiently.

CROSS TRAINING

The nerves that carry sensation from each limb to the spine connect with nerves carrying sensations down into the opposite limb. Because of this, exercising one limb will improve muscular function in its mate. In fact, exercising the legs can cause changes to occur in the arms. This is because exercising the lower limbs induces systemic effects (heart, liver, blood) that increase performance in the upper limbs. However, exercising the arms has little effect on the legs because the arm musculature is relatively small compared to that of the legs.

Muscle fibers enlarge in response to demand. A muscle will enlarge if it is contracted long enough, often enough, and hard enough. It will do this without hormones, and for a while even without protein in the diet, because it gets preferential access to amino acids and utilizes available protein in the body for muscle synthesis.

EASTERN EXERCISES

Eastern exercise techniques have become very popular. Tai-chi is a very relaxing exercise that involves the performance of slow, formalized dancelike movements. It is a relaxation technique that has a meditative quality. It has appeal for people of all ages and can be done almost anywhere. Tai-chi combines deep breathing, relaxation, and slow, gentle, structured movement. Chinese martial artist Chang San Feng developed Tai-chi more than 700 years ago as a method of self-defense for monks. Since then it has evolved into an art that exercises the body and mind.

Tai-chi literally means "moving life force." Its choreographed movements, called *forms*, resemble a slow, graceful dance. The movements were designed to mimic animal movements, such as those of the snake and the white crane. Tai-chi is based on the Taoist belief that good health results from balanced *chi*, or life force. In accordance with this belief, the forms are practiced in order to stimulate and balance the body's chi. This is done through proper breathing and by learning to keep the muscles active but relaxed, the mind alert but calm, and body movements slow but well-coordinated.

A goal of Tai-chi is to enhance body awareness (proprioception) and overall well-being. It is claimed that Tai-chi has healing benefits that include boosting the immune system, improving digestion, decreasing depression and anxiety, and promoting relaxation. Recent research involving older adults has produced evidence that Tai-chi can help improve balance and lower blood pressure. This can lead to significant reduction in falls (almost 50% in one study), which is thought to be due to improved proprioception, joint mobility, and strength. Because aerobic exercise is the best exercise for the heart, Tai-chi generally should be practiced along with, rather than in place of, regular moderate aerobic exercise. Tai-chi is safe. Students are taught to recognize and maintain stable footing until they develop a firm "root," or ability to balance. The movements of Tai-chi are less jarring than those of a low-impact exercise class. In several studies involving rheumatoid arthritis patients, those who practiced Tai-chi for 10 weeks had no increase in joint symptoms when compared with patients who were not involved in Tai-chi training.

Tai-chi classes can be found at health clubs, hospitals, martial arts schools, and community centers. Videos are also available, but there is no substitute for hands-on instruction for feedback and for realizing the full potential of Tai-chi. To find out more about the health benefits of Tai-chi, you can contact the American Tai-chi for Health Association, 26895 Aliso Creek Rd., Suite B-101, Aliso Viejo, CA 92656; 949/422-2577.

Yoga exercises are a very pleasant way of stretching, relaxing, and meditating—all at the same time. The various positions—called *asanas*—generally stretch and relax the body. Proper breathing techniques are important during these exercises. Source materials are books and videotapes. Although it is possible to teach yourself yoga, it usually is better to join a class at your local health club or community center to get started and then carry on by yourself after you learn the basics.

Tae-bo combines Eastern martial art techniques with aerobic exercises. It provides a rigorous workout. Videotapes are available for rental or purchase.

SPECIAL TECHNIQUES

Special exercising techniques such as the *Alexander method*, which emphasizes balance of body segments, or the *Feldenkrais* technique, directed toward balancing the right against the left side of the body by correcting the imbalance caused by handedness, are available as physical therapy treatment when indicated for special postural problems.

Isokinetic exercise using special machines that progressively load a joint through its arc of movement is prescribed for special athletic training. More details on fitness, including illustrated instructions for specific exercises, can be found in my book, *All About Bone: An Owner's Manual* (Demos, 1998).

It has been said that exercise is to the body what reading is to the mind, and I hope I have convinced you of its benefits by now. An interesting bit of trivia is that you exercise 45 facial muscles by frowning, and it takes only the risorius and zygomaticus muscles in tandem with 15 other muscles in the face to smile, and the average person has only 15 laughs a day. I am not suggesting that you stop smiling and frown instead just to exercise your face. By all means, keep smiling. Just smile more often. And a program of regular exercise should help you do just that.

QUESTIONS AND ANSWERS

Exercise

Q: What is the Pilates exercise system? How does it differ from other programs?

A: The Pilates (Pi-LAH-teez) method was developed during World War I by Joseph Hubertus. Pilates, a German-born boxer who was fascinated with fitness. The method emphasizes precision of movement, which focuses and exercises the mind as well as the body. The exercise is low-impact in nature, designed to build a person's "core" by strengthening the abdomen, lower back, and buttocks. Pilates was popularized by the New York City Ballet because of the exercise program's ability to build strength and flexibility through twisting, stretching, and balancing, without adding bulky muscles. Many celebrities, including Madonna, have endorsed the system. Pilates studios have sprung up all over the United States and abroad. Pilates classes must be supervised by someone properly trained in the method.

Q: What equipment is it necessary to have to exercise properly?

A: Very little. Light weights and elastic bands can be purchased inexpensively at a local sporting goods store.

Stationary bicycles, weight benches, treadmills, Stairmasters, and Nordic ski equipment are available for those who want to have a gym at home. Fancier equipment, including Nautilus-type machines designed to provide resistance exercise for specific muscle groups, are usually found in health clubs.

Q: Why is it so important to decrease your body fat?

A: Looks aside, each pound of body fat needs approximately one mile of blood vessels for its support. Too many extra pounds can place considerable extra strain on your heart and lungs to support this extra tissue.

Q: Are there any absolute contraindications to exercise training?

A: Yes, there are. These include heart block or congestive heart failure, unstable angina or uncontrolled cardiac arrhythmia, serious electrocardiographic changes, or a recent heart attack.

Contraindications to an exercise program might include chronic cardiac disease, uncontrolled metabolic disease, and uncontrolled high blood pressure.

Q: Who gets the greatest benefit from exercise?

A: The U.S. Census Bureau has projected that by the year 2010 more than half of all Americans will be older than 35 years of age, with 25 percent 55 years of age and older. Older people who have appropriately active lifestyles seem to get the greatest benefit from exercise, particularly when one "goes from doing nothing to doing something."

Q: How much aerobic exercise is required to produce significant health benefits?

A: Not much. You need only a cumulative total of 30 to 50 minutes of aerobic exercise a day performed for three to five days a week and one set of resistance exercises targeting major muscle groups performed twice a week to produce significant health benefit. The aerobic part need not be a structured activity. It can be satisfied through regular participation in many common physical tasks, such as housekeeping, walking, gardening, and the like.

Q: If an active lifestyle correlates with long life and is important for physical and mental well-being, why don't people exercise more?

A: There are a lot of excuses, but I suppose the bottom line is that with modern transportation and home entertainment they don't have to, it's easier not to, so they don't. Because of this, physical inactivity remains a significant health care problem in the United States. Fewer than 40 percent of adults engage in vigorous exercise on a regular basis, and 25 percent of adults are almost totally inactive. This pattern of inactivity starts very early in life. A study questioning children about their activities over the previous two weeks revealed that only 50 percent of school-aged children had engaged in strenuous physical activities. There was an almost 50 percent reduction in enrollment in physical education classes in the United States between 1991 and 1995.

Q: Can seniors successfully participate in competitive athletics?

A: Examination of records from Masters athletic competitions reveals that the decline in physical activities for Masters athletes is gradual and the potential for seniors to participate in competitive athletics can persist well into the seventh decade of life.

Q: What ultimately determines the strength gains possible in older adults?

A: The age-related reduction in the number of spinal nerve cells, which begins before age 65, is the ultimate determinant of strength gains possible in older adults.

Q: Do aging muscles utilize oxygen normally?

A: Maximum oxygen utilization is an accurate measurement of the level of athletic fitness. Maximum oxygen utilization declines by up to 15 percent every 10 years after age 25. This most probably is due to associated changes in the function of the heart and blood vessels. However, an endurance exercise program throughout life can reduce this rate of decline by 50 percent.

Q: How does "metabolic" fitness differ from "athletic" fitness?

A: "Metabolic" fitness is a reduction of risk factors that predispose a person to diabetes and cardiovascular disease. "Athletic" fitness refers to an increase in maximum oxygen uptake. The quantity (intensity times frequency) of exercise required to achieve improvement in metabolic fitness is substantially less than that necessary to improve athletic fitness. For example, exercise to maintain cardiorespiratory fitness requires only a training intensity of raising your heart rate to 60 to 90 percent of its maximum for a duration of 30 to 60 minutes (this can be intermittent) for three to five days per week (training more than five days a week adds no additional benefit). Such a program should be tailored to the individual depending on his initial level of fitness.

Q: What are some of the risk factors for activity-related injury?

A: Such risk factors include osteoarthritis, weakness, restriction of joint motion, joint deformity, previous obesity, and previous joint injury.

Q: Just how important is exercise for children?

A: Many people believe that although inactivity is widespread in adults, children are naturally active and that the health risks associated with a sedentary lifestyle, such as diabetes and heart disease, are far more pressing in adults. This is not necessarily true. According to the Surgeon General's report on physical activity and health, activity levels decline as a child matures and drop dramatically when he/she enters adolescence. Almost half of American young people ages 10 to 20 are not regularly vigorously active, and 64 percent of Americans between the ages of 6 and 17 cannot pass a basic fitness test.

A child's exercise program should be tailored to his age and needs. Children up to 5 years of age are just learning fundamental skills; from 5 to 10 a child can begin to coordinate moves related to actual sports; from 10 on her or she can master the complex motor skills required and has the cognitive ability to learn strategies for adult forms of most sports. Safety, of course, is paramount, and a prudent approach will minimize overuse injuries and more serious trauma (55 percent of all playground injuries occur on the monkey bars).

Although Tiger Woods was playing nine holes of golf by age 3 and Chris Evert took up tennis at 5, the same age as Olympic medalist Shannon Miller began her gymnastic career, the American Academy of Pediatrics recommends that youngsters be discouraged from single sport specialization before adolescence. The risks include physical and psychological damage such as repetitive strain injuries, stress fractures, eating disorders, delayed menstruation, emotional stress, and burnout. Waiting to specialize until age 13, a child is more physically and emotionally mature. This helps ensure that he or she is pursuing an activity that really interests him or her rather than just fulfilling the dream of a coach or parent.

Regular exercise is an important strategy to maintain health for children in adolescence. It helps strengthen bones, facilitates weight control, and can lessen cardiovascular risk factors. A child's mental health benefits and an active childhood lays the groundwork for a lifetime of fitness.

Q: What dietary suggestions do you have for the older athlete?

A: The senior athlete should make sure to get enough daily carbohydrates and protein to sustain weight and energy. Vitamins are important, especially vitamins C and E. These antioxidants help the body neutralize unstable free radicals, compounds that accumulate in our immune systems as we age and destroy healthy cells. A daily dose of 500 to 3,000 mg of vitamin C, 400 to 800 International Units of vitamin E, and 400 mcg of selenium should be sufficient. Garlic is also a potent antioxidant. You can buy odorless supplements.

Some fat is necessary in the diet. Unsaturated fats help the body retain B-complex vitamins and decrease the effects of stress. Such fats also maintain cell membrane integrity and help fight off the invasion of cancer cells. Cold-water fish (tuna, sardines, salmon) and nuts (especially walnuts) with omega-3 fats discourage heart disease.

The antiaging athlete's diet should include at least eight vegetables and fruits a day, minimally processed foods, beans at least several times a week, and at least eight glasses of water a day.

Food should be enjoyed and supplements should be taken responsibly. Small meals (particularly at dinner) and frequent light snacks (grazing) during the day are better for you than three heavy meals.

If overweight is a problem, dieting alone is not effective as a method of permanent weight loss. People who eat less than their bodies require regain all the weight they have lost plus some extra weight for good measure, within three to five years of dieting. A recent weight loss study observed three groups. The first group exercised and dieted. The second group dieted but did not exercise. The third group exercised but did not diet. As you might imagine, the combined diet and exercise group lost the most weight. Those who dieted without exercising were in the middle, and those who only exercised lost the least amount of weight. However, a surprising thing occurred in the second year of the study. The group that only exercised regained very little of the weight they lost. On the other hand, the group that had dieted and exercised gained back more than 50 percent of what they had lost, while those who dieted without exercising gained back what they had lost plus a few pounds more.

Granted, exercise is a slow way to lose weight, but it may be the wisest method of weight management in view of the extra benefits it often brings. These include increased energy, stress relief, and a boost in self-esteem that leaves people happier with their fit bodies and less concerned about the number on the scale.

Q: What controls the ultimate athletic performance a human being can achieve?

A: Lions can sprint up to 50 mph, and cheetahs move even faster, flooring it to a sizzling 70 mph. Most humans have trouble running 25 mph. It wasn't until 1959 that Roger Bannister, Britain's running doc, ran the mile in less than four minutes, coming in .06 of a second under the charmed figure. Many four-minute or less miles have been run since then, but less than 17 additional seconds have been shaved off Bannister's record, about a third of a second per year.

Better training and equipment account for most of the improvement, but shoes and diet can get only so good before runners hit a wall. What slows the human body down is the chemistry of its muscles. The key to speed is making muscles contract faster, and the key to that is providing as much oxygen as possible. Approximately 80 percent of the energy used to run a mile comes directly from oxygen.

Oxygen is processed through the cellular components known as the mitochondria (from the Greek *mitos* = thread and *khondros* = grain), which are the power plants of the cells. Human mitochondria take up only about 3 percent of the space in a cell. However, mitochondria are far larger in animals that run the fastest. The mitochondria of an antelope, which can easily run a two-minute mile, are three times larger than ours.

Genetic engineering may provide the answer. A benign virus has already been equipped with genetic material that codes for muscle growth. Mice injected with this virus quickly increase muscle bulk up to 20 percent, becoming not only bigger but also stronger. If humans could be genetically engineered to have more mitochondria, bigger hearts, and more blood vessels, they might run about 40 mph. Runners are not the only athletes who would benefit by this kind of genetic redesign. Baseball players could increase their bat speed so that home runs could fly hundreds of feet farther. Boosting leg strength in a football kicker would enable a 75 to 90 yard field goal.

Whether such superperformance would be good for the athlete is another question. Racehorses, which are bred and trained for speeds they were not designed to run, suffer all types of physical damage as a result of overuse, from fractured legs to bleeding lungs. You might see the same thing in a human being when normal anatomy is subjected to excessive strain.

Finally, there is the moral question of developing athletic excellence through tricky genetics rather than because of skill and will. It is doubtful indeed that such metabolic manipulations will contribute anything of enduring value to the field of competitive athletics.

Q: What is the best advice for winter conditioning for spring sports?

A: First of all, don't do too much too fast. Start off at only 25 to 50 percent of what you were doing the previous summer. One of the most common mistakes athletes make is failing to load up on water the night before an extended period of activity. Drink at least one quart of water. This will help replace the 54 ounces of body fluid lost on average per hour of exercise through perspiration in hot weather. You will know you have had enough when your urine runs clear. This can help avoid cramps due to dehydration. Warmup exercises and sport-specific stretches are essential before, between, and after vigorous exercise. Being in shape is important even for nonaerobic sports such as golf. Low back exercises are useful for golf, tennis, skating, and baseball. Balance training helps tennis and blading. Leg exercises are valuable for all sports, particularly running and biking. Tennis players should balance their workouts on both sides of their bodies, not just the side of the racquet arm. The best advice? Stay fit all year long.

Q: How do you stay motivated for exercise?

A: First, you should choose an exercise that suits your personality or mood of the day. If you are competitive, choose a competitive sport. If you have a strong work ethic, do household tasks or gardening with vigor. If you are very social in nature, you can try mall-walking, join a gym, or exercise with others. If you are strongly goal-oriented, engage in traditional fitness activities. Lift more, run faster and further, and so forth. If you are a loner, take a long walk, hike a trail, or try Eastern-style exercise. If you enjoy playful activity, try horseback riding, ice skating, skiing, or dancing. If you are a couch potato, just make a commitment to do *something*, no matter what, every day. Walk even a few blocks or climb a few stairs.

Some rules to follow are:

1. Rethink exercise. You don't always have to exhaust yourself.
2. Take a breather. You occasionally need to do less, and that's all right.
3. Develop the habit of exercise. It takes weeks to do this, so keep at it.
4. Reserve a time for regular exercise, and don't let anything interfere.
5. Let everyone know what your exercise time is and insist on not being disturbed.

6. Be patient with yourself. Some days you may be more motivated than others.
7. Don't let others discourage you.
8. Team up with others if you can. This will help your motivation.
9. Plan ahead and be prepared to exercise.
10. Set achievable goals, and you will be rewarded with your accomplishment.
11. Affirm your efforts because this will inspire you to continue.
12. Customize your approach to exercise to make it more enjoyable.
13. Be constantly aware of your body. If you feel in any way uncomfortable, change your routine.
14. Finally, complement your exercise with a well-balanced diet, get adequate sleep, and reduce unhealthy influences such as stress and smoking.

Q: Can exercise increase balance and prevent falling in the elderly?

A: One-third of those over age 35 will fall each year, and up to 15 percent of those falls may cause serious injury. Up to 50 percent of elderly people report fear of falling after a fall, and they often restrict their activity as a result. Actually, children and young adults fall more often than the elderly because they are more active. In the elderly, most falls are the result of trips, slips, or momentary loss of balance. Approximately 15 percent of falls involve fainting, seizures, or acute illnesses such as stroke. For the first two weeks after a hospital stay, elderly patients are at more than four times the risk of falling than they are some three months later.

The ability to restore one's bearing following a challenge such as tripping over an obstacle is called dynamic balance. This ability declines with age, especially following a stroke or in people with Parkinson's disease. When dynamic balance deteriorates, a person's reflexes may be slowed and weight-bearing sensations from his legs may be diminished. The result is relying more on vision to ensure stability. If vision is also impaired, it makes it difficult to make effective compensations for being pulled off balance in time to avoid a fall.

Research confirms that older and more frail people are at an increased risk of falling. Long-acting sedatives such as Valium, antiseizure drugs, and antidepressant medications may also increase the risk of falling. Anyone who has fallen twice or more in one year or who needs to use his or her hands to rise from a chair of normal height runs a double risk to that of a population of not at risk similarly aged individuals. The higher a person's peril of falling, the higher the chance of serious injury.

Balance exercise programs have been able to reduce falls by up to 25 percent. A home visit by an occupational therapist to identify home hazards, such as throw rugs, improper footwear, lack of bath mats, and the like, can reduce falls in the group at risk by as much as 30 percent. When used for a year or more, various medications for osteoporosis have cut the number of hip fracture incidents in half. Also, specially designed padding at the hips, known as hip protectors, can immediately cut the danger of hip fracture from a fall by 50 percent.

Because many factors contribute to falling, each individual at high risk deserves thorough evaluation. Treatment must address as many factors as possible, and focus should be placed on the improvement of balance and safety.

Now we are ready to take a look at your joints, one by one. So, let's start with the deepest joint in the body, the one that enables our upright posture, but in doing so is subject to the vicissitudes of disease, injury, and aging. I refer, of course, to the hip.

4

The Hip

ANATOMY

Although the knee is the largest joint in the body, the hip is the
deepest joint. The hip is a ball-and-socket joint, much like the
glenohumeral (shoulder) joint. In contrast to the shoulder,
which is very shallow (similar to a ball in a saucer) and sacrifices stability for range of motion, the hip (like a ball in a teacup)
is considerably deeper, relinquishing range of motion for much-
needed stability.

Two bones participate in the hip joint. The "ball" is the end
of the femur (thigh bone) and fits into the *acetabulum* (from the
Latin "little vinegar dish") or hip socket, which is part of the
pelvis. The upper part of the femur has a short, angled "neck"
upon which the ball sits. The angles (both forward and sideways) of this neck and the inclination (both forward and down)
of the hip socket allow required motion while providing maximum positional stability.

All joints in the body are lever systems that maximize muscle function (Figure 4-1a, b). The hip is a first-degree lever,
much like a seesaw. The fulcrum of this lever is at the center of
the joint. Those muscles that move the hip to the side provide
the force, and the leg is the weight to be lifted. Bone is arrayed
within the head and neck in the femur to construct stress lines

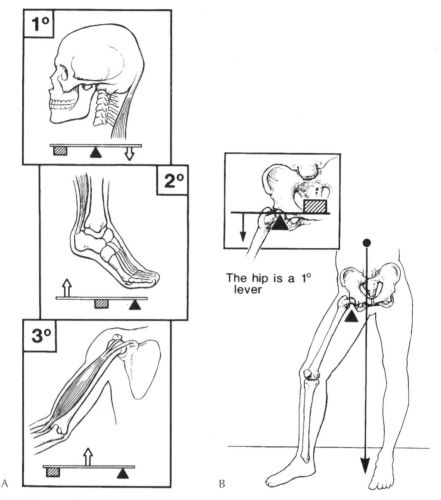

FIGURE 4-1   Lever systems.

that maximize bony resistance to superimposed strain. This adaptation of the inner structure of the bone to mechanical requirements related to load can be seen in all of your joints.

Like your other joints, the hip is surrounded by a fibrous capsule consisting of a number of *ligaments*. The cavity of the socket is deepened by a fibrocartilaginous rim, and further stability is provided through a thick band of tissue called the *ligamentum teres* (smooth cylindrical ligament), which attaches the apex of the head to the middle of the socket. The hip is a diarthrosis (joint containing fluid) and therefore is lined with an extensive synovial membrane. The fluid secreted by this membrane provides lubrication and nourishment to the articular cartilage of the hip (Figure 4-2).

Thirteen muscles enable extensive movement of the hip. It can flex (bend), extend (straighten), adduct (move toward the midline of the body), abduct (move from the midline of the body), circumduct (move in a circle), and rotate (twist in or out). Some of the strongest muscles in the body activate the hip. The power that enables track and field athletes to run and jump and major league batters to hit home runs comes from the hips.

Hip problems can be different in children and adults. Let's characterize them.

CHILDREN

Hip problems are common in children and have the potential to cause considerable disability throughout the rest of life. Three factors significantly contribute to the seriousness of disorders of the hip in children:

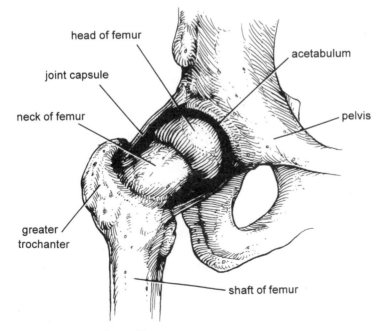

FIGURE 4-2   Anatomy of your hip.

1. *Delay in diagnosis.* The hip joint is the deepest joint in the body compared with other joints such as the wrist or the ankle. Because of this, physical diagnosis is more of a problem. Furthermore, the obturator nerve innervates (provides a nerve supply) both the hip and the area on the inside of the knee. For this reason, hip disorders may present only with knee pain. This can contribute to a delay in diagnosis.

2. *Anatomic status.* Because of increasing longevity and the effect of standing upright, the hip is subject to degenerative arthritis, even in normal individuals, but particularly in those who have had childhood hip disease or injury. This is because of overuse and the effect that upright posture has on focusing the load-bearing area in a ball-and-socket joint.

3. *Tenuous blood supply.* The vessels to the hip are few in number and are vulnerable to inflammation, infection, or injury. They even can be stretched and compressed by certain positions of the head of the femur in the joint.

Workup

In the child, a thorough evaluation of the hip is important because of vulnerability of the hip joint to damage. Is there a family history of hip problems? Some of the more common hip disorders in childhood (e.g., congenital dislocation) occur in families. Has the child complained of pain? Is a limp apparent? Are there other signs of illness? An examination of the hips is conducted, assessing range of motion and any tenderness present, as well as imaging, which may include ultrasound, computed tomography (CT) scanning, or magnetic resonance imaging (MRI).

Laboratory studies include a complete blood count and an erythrocyte sedimentation rate (a laboratory blood test that can indicate inflammation) to rule out infection. When an *effusion* (accumulation of fluid or blood in a joint) is suspected, the hip joint can be aspirated (fluid drawn out through a needle).

The causes of hip pain are numerous. The process usually can be differentiated from the history, physical examination, laboratory studies, and imaging.

Infection of the Hip

Infection of the hip is a surgical emergency that requires immediate drainage to avoid the consequences of septic (infectious) arthritis, which may destroy the entire joint.

Avascular Necrosis

Avascular necrosis is death of bone at the head of the femur. This condition may be associated with trauma, infections, the administration of steroid drugs, and certain systemic disorders that cause hip degeneration, including Gaucher's disease, lupus, sickle cell disease, and other blood disorders. The common idiopathic (cause not known) form of avascular necrosis is called Perthes' disease.

Transient Synovitis

Transient *synovitis* is a mild inflammation of the hip joint lining that occurs in children. It is also known as irritable hip. The cause is not known, but in many patients an upper respiratory infection precedes the onset of hip pain.

Transient synovitis must be differentiated from septic arthritis of the hip. It can be managed with rest. A more serious condition such as septic arthritis or Perthes' disease should be considered if it does not resolve in short order.

Developmental Hip Dysplasia

The arms are considerably more functionally advanced at birth than are the legs. A newborn reflexively grasps objects tightly with his or her hands, but the underdeveloped legs are maintained in the fetal position bent upward and strongly resist straightening. The hip socket is small relative to the size of the femoral head, which renders the hip unstable and at risk for slipping out.

Developmental *dysplasia* of the hip (DDH) includes a spectrum of anatomic abnormalities of the hip that may be present at birth or may develop during infancy. These conditions cover such mild faults as a shallow acetabulum to severe defects such as complete hip dislocation. The earlier the diagnosis is made, the greater the chance of successful treatment. A positive family history; breech (feet first) position at birth; and the presence of other orthopaedic problems, such as wry (twisted) neck or foot or knee deformities, place the hip at greater risk for DDH. Examination of the hip at birth can demonstrate hip instability. When suspicion is high, ultrasound imaging will confirm the diagnosis. Radiographs become progressively more reliable for diagnosis as the child grows.

Management of the infant with DDH is with any of a number of splints or harnesses that hold the head in the socket so that normal growth of the head and deepening of the socket can proceed. Traction or reduction (relocation of the femoral head into the hip socket) with application of a spica (figure-of-eight) cast are other alternatives. Soft tissue obstruction to reduction may be present and can be confirmed by an arthrogram (X-ray after injection of radiopaque dye into the hip joint). Complications include avascular necrosis and recurrent dislocation.

Surgery for resistant cases or older patients in whom diagnosis has been delayed includes a variety of procedures to provide a bony shelf for support, deepen the acetabulum, or increase its angulation or that of the femoral neck so that the head of the femur will fit securely in its socket.

Legg-Calvé-Perthes Disease

Legg-Calvé-Perthes (LCP) disease is also known as *coxa plana* (flattened femoral head). Its cause is not known, but a variation in the blood supply to the femoral head may be inherited as a predisposing factor. Whereas congenital dislocation of the hip occurs more frequently in girls, LCP is seen more frequently in boys between the ages of 4 and 8 years. Approximately 10 percent of cases involve both hips, with a brief time interval between the onset on each side. Physical examination reveals a painful limp and lack of hip rotation. The condition is classified by the extent of head involvement and the stage of hip degeneration. Anywhere from a small portion of the head to the entire head can be involved. Degeneration of the hip is divided into four stages: (1) synovitis, (2) bony collapse, (3) bony fragmentation, and (4) reconstitution. Conservative treatment involves bracing to "contain" the hip in the socket and in some cases to avoid the pressure of weight bearing. Surgery sometimes may be necessary to reposition the femoral head directly into the acetabulum.

Management must be tailored to each child's needs because healing of the hip may require several years of treatment.

Slipped Capital Femoral Epiphysis

The growth zone at the juncture of the neck and head of the femur (capital femoral physis) is vulnerable to weakening and slipping. The majority of children with this condition are obese. Obesity contributes to overloading of the hip and mechanical slipping at the growth plate, which occurs when the mechanical stresses exceed its strength. The hip is anatomically vulnerable because of its biomechanics. Pressure across the joint on weight bearing can be as high as four times body weight. The growth plate is weaker than other skeletal components during puberty, which makes it easy for slipped capital femoral epiphysis to occur.

The slip may be acute (sudden) or chronic (gradual). The child complains of thigh or knee pain and has a painful limp. Physical examination reveals loss of hip rotation. Diagnosis usually can be made by conventional X-ray examination that includes a good lateral (side) view of the hip. The objective of treatment is to stabilize the growth plate to prevent further slippage. This requires an operation with metallic (usually screw) fixation. For severe slips, an osteotomy (cutting with repositioning) of the hip is required to correct the deformity.

Chondrolysis (degeneration of the articular cartilage) and avascular necrosis can occur as complications to slipped capital femoral epiphysis.

Now let's take a look at ...

THE ADULT HIP

Bursitis

Common benign (not serious) conditions that affect the adult hip include bursitis and tendinitis. There are many *bursae* associated with the hip region whose function is to reduce friction between adjacent soft tissue structures or between tendon and bone. Bursae are small sacs that have a lining similar to synovial membrane and are vulnerable to a variety of irritating conditions.

Repetitive stress on a bursa can produce an inflammatory response. The trochanteric bursa, located over the side of the hip, is vulnerable to stress such as that imposed by jogging on the camber of a road or with flat feet. You may have a bursitis if you have pain over the side of your hip that extends down your thigh and tenderness on deep pressure over the upper outer portion of the thigh. Treatment includes rest, ice, a nonsteroidal antiinflammatory drug (NSAID, such as ibuprofen, Naprosyn, etc.), and correction of an inept running style. Aspiration with injection of Novocain and a corticosteroid drug may be indicated.

Snapping hip is closely associated with the trochanteric bursa. You experience a snapping sound on certain movements of the hip that may or may not be accompanied by pain. The snap is caused by a tendinous or fascial band, such as the tensor fascia lata, slipping over the bone on the outside of the hip. Stretching exercises for this band are usually prescribed. Surgical release may be necessary.

Tendinitis

Tendinitis (inflammation of a tendon) and muscle tears can occur with repeated trauma. Treatment is with rest, ice, compression, and antiinflammatory medication. Surgical repair may be required for a complete rupture.

Hamstring strain or muscle tear is common. Buttock pain referred down the leg caused by a tight muscle (usually the piriformis) compressing the sciatic nerve also can occur.

Fractures

Why do so many older people break their hips? Osteoporosis (brittle bones), a disease particularly common in postmenopausal women, weakens the bones by making them more porous. This makes fractures more likely, particularly in the hip, which, as one of the largest weight-bearing joints of the body, is under severe stress during standing and walking.

Most hip fractures occur at the base (intertrochanteric area) of the hip. Fractures that occur across the neck of the hip (transcervical fractures) may interrupt circulation to the femoral head. A break across the upper shaft of the femur bone as it becomes the hip (subtrochanteric fracture) is the least common.

Diagnosis usually is not a problem except in the case of an incomplete or impacted fracture, in which the broken ends of the bone are jammed into each other. A history of a fall in an older person, with pain, often severe, as well as deformity (usually shortening and rolling out of the leg), abnormal motion, and a positive X-ray, will clinch the diagnosis of a fractured hip.

Treatment

Almost all hip fractures are treated surgically. A fracture across the neck of the bone often can be fixed with threaded pins introduced under fluoroscopic control. In patients over age 65 in whom the blood supply to the femoral head is at severe risk, a prosthesis may be used to replace the hip. Intertrochanteric fractures at the base of the hip can be treated with one of a variety of metal hip compression screws held in a plate that is screwed to the shaft of the bone. If the shaft itself is broken, a metal nail may be inserted into the central canal of the femur to hold the broken pieces in place. A compression screw helps the bone edges heal.

Physical therapy is started immediately after surgery. Gradual weight bearing with the use of a walking aid (walker or crutches progressing to a cane) is an important part of rehabilitation. As in any pelvic surgery, the use of blood-thinning medication is advisable to avoid the complication of blood clots in the pelvis or legs.

Arthritis

The hip is frequently affected by arthritis because it is one of the major weight-bearing joints of the body. Both osteoarthritis and rheumatoid arthritis (see Chapter 2) can involve the hip. The patient suffers pain and complains of stiffness in the joint. He or she begins to walk with a painful limp. Motion of the joint is limited and painful. X-rays and special examinations of the blood confirm the diagnosis.

Treatment consists of the application of heat or ice, the use of a cane to unload the hip during walking, and an oral antiinflammatory medication, usually an NSAID. Cox-2 inhibitors, a new class of drugs that, while inhibiting enzymes that destroy joint cartilage, have a minimal irritating effect on the gastrointestinal

Stretching Exercises

A. *Leg scissors.* Lie relaxed on your back. Spread legs as far apart as possible, keeping knees straight. Bring legs back together again.

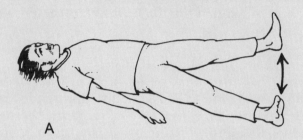

B. *Leg rotations.* Lie relaxed on your back. Straighten right leg and bend left leg. Pointing toes of right foot toward the ceiling, rotate the right leg clockwise and then counter-clockwise. Now straighten left leg and bend right knee. Repeat the exercise with left leg.

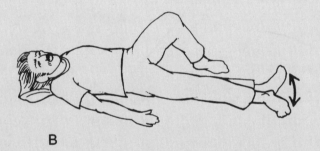

C. *Knee crossover stretch.* Lie as illustrated on your right side. Straighten your legs. Bend your left knee up to your chest. Cross left knee over right leg, down toward supporting surface. Now lift left knee and return to starting position. Roll over and repeat exercise with right leg.

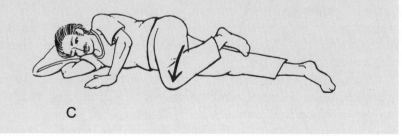

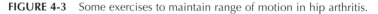

FIGURE 4-3   Some exercises to maintain range of motion in hip arthritis.

Strengthening Exercises

D. *Side lifts.* Lay on right side as illustrated. Keep left leg straight and in line with your body. Lift it as high as you can. Hold for a count of 6, then lower slowly. Roll over to left side and perform exercise with right leg.

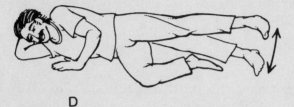

D

E. *Lifting knee-to-chest.* Lie on yourback as illustrated. Bend right leg at the hip and bring the knee to your chest. Lower the leg slowly to its starting position. Relax. Repeat exercise with left leg.

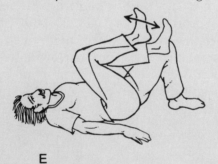

E

F. *Straight leg lifts.* Lie flat on your back. Keeping left knee bent, straightn right knee and lift leg as high as you can. Lower leg slowly to the floor. Repeat exercise with left leg.

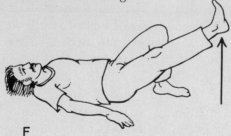

F

All of these exercises should be performed slowly, trying for maximum stretch or lift. Start with 2–5 repetitions and work up to a maximum of 25–30.

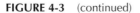

FIGURE 4-3   (continued)

tract, are becoming popular in the conservative management of arthritis. Physical therapy, including exercise, is often prescribed. When arthritis strikes one or both hips, performing even the simplest tasks can be difficult and painful. It is therefore important to stretch and strengthen the muscles that control joint movements. The following exercises will help maintain range of motion of the hips (Fig. 4-3).

Surgery

Surgical treatment of an arthritic hip includes (1) *osteotomy*, an operation in which cutting and/or wedging the bone allows the surgeon to reposition the hip in its socket; (2) *arthrodesis* (fusion), where the joint is fixed in a functional position so that painful movement is no longer possible; and (3) *total joint replacement*.

The rate of total hip replacement is 280 per 100,000 population in people 65 and older. In 1998, 250,000 primary and revision total hip replacements were performed in the United States, of which 59 percent were performed on women. That number is expected to increase by 10 percent by the year 2002. The average charge for this procedure in the United States was $20,290—with hospital charges accounting for 73 percent of the costs (mean hospital stay was four days). The average surgeon's fee in the United States was $5,450. Approximately 30,000 hip revision surgeries are performed each year in the United States. These surgeries are more difficult to perform, place patients at greater risk for blood loss and infection, cost more than the first hip replacement, and require a longer hospital stay.

The procedure of total hip replacement has been refined to the point where it has become almost a routine operation on the orthopaedic agenda. The first joint arthroplasty (creation of an artificial joint) was not performed on the hip but on the jaw. In 1840 Garnochan, from New York, placed a wooden block between the resected ends of an ankylosed (fused) temporomandibular (jaw) joint. Subsequently, various other biologic and foreign materials were used, such as skin, muscle, fascia, pig bladder, and gold foil. The earliest documented total hip replacement was performed by Theophilus Gluck, a German surgeon, who in 1891 replaced a diseased hip with an ivory ball and socket, which he screwed into place. This hip dislocated almost immediately on weight bearing. In 1933 Marion Smith-Petersen introduced mold arthroplasty (Gr. arthro = joint, plasty = to form). His original design was bell-shaped and made of glass. The idea was to stimulate cartilage regeneration on the femoral head. Subsequently, Pyrex, Bakelite, and finally Vitallium, a cobalt-chromium alloy were used. The late Sir John Charnley, a contemporary English orthopaedic surgeon, pioneered in the development of materials and techniques for modern total joint replacement.

The technique of total joint replacement involves implanting a device that resurfaces and replaces the degenerative articular surfaces of the hip. Artificial total joints are composed of a hard plastic (polyethylene) portion matched with a metallic component, usually an alloy of cobalt, chrome, and titanium or stainless steel. The components of a total hip are cemented into the joint after it is prepared to receive them by removing the head of the femur and the articular cartilage in the acetabulum, reaming the femoral channel, and deepening and shaping the hip socket. Joint replacements that do not require cement but rely on bony ingrowth into a specially treated metal surface incorporating metal beads or fibers have been developed and are increasingly used and preferred in younger patients. Currently, "metal-on-metal" implants have been approved by the U.S. Food and Drug Administration and are entering the market. Whereas the plastic and metal implant has a life expectancy of 15 to 20 years depending on the patient's weight and activity (it usually is the plastic that wears out), these new metal-on-metal prostheses could allow the patient to be reasonably active and still last 30 years or more. A patient could not run a marathon, but activities such as biking, vigorous walking, and doubles tennis would be acceptable.

Overtaxing an implant is not without consequences. For example, former professional football and baseball player Bo Jackson dislocated his hip in 1992, developed severe arthritis, and had a type of total hip replacement. He went back to playing baseball and in 1995 had a revision. A few years later, he required yet another revision as a result of overactivity.

Operative risks include blood clots and pneumonia. Infection also may occur. This can be superficial or deep and may be evident during the hospital stay or even several years afterward. Superficial infections can be treated locally, but deep infections may require further surgery for drainage or even removal of the prosthesis. Because spread of infection from another part of the body can occur, people who have had total joint replacements are given prophylactic antibiotics before dental work (including cleaning the teeth) or other types of surgery. Late complications include loosening of the prosthesis, which may require replacement; dislocation, which usually is treated by relocation and the temporary use of a brace; wear of the metal and plastic joint surfaces that can result in irritation of surrounding tissue from worn metal or plastic particles, contributing to loosening; breakage, requiring a second operation for replacement of the broken component; and damage to nerves or vessels in the area of surgery, resulting in temporary or permanent weakness or numbness in the leg.

Ambulation with limited weight bearing is started immediately after surgery. Hospital recovery usually is brief. Most people can handle their tasks of daily living with increased facility and enjoy a more independent, mobile lifestyle after total hip replacement. However, the artificial joint does not have the biologic capacity of normal tissue and cannot be subjected to excessive stresses or strains. Nonetheless, most total hip replacement patients can participate in most of the activities they took part in before their surgery if they are careful. This includes sex (Fig 4-4).

The main benefit to the patient after total hip replacement is pain relief, which may be dramatic. Soreness can persist because of surgery, as well as weakness in the muscles surrounding the hip joint. Muscle power, lost because the painful, arthritic joint was not used, usually returns with exercise when pain is relieved. Motion of the joint generally will improve.

Postoperative care includes supervised exercise. Living changes at home, such as rearranging furniture to make it easier to get around and correcting hazards that may lead to accidents, are recommended.

A. Face to face (bottom position is safe for patient with joint replacement)

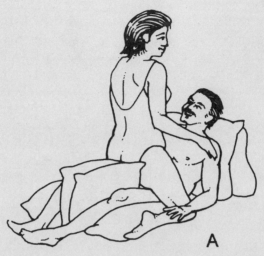

B. Sitting (either position is safe for patient with joint replacement)

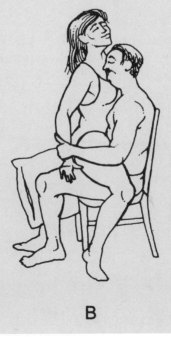

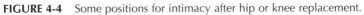

FIGURE 4-4   Some positions for intimacy after hip or knee replacement.

C. Man kneeling—woman lying (safe for woman with hip or knee joint replacement)

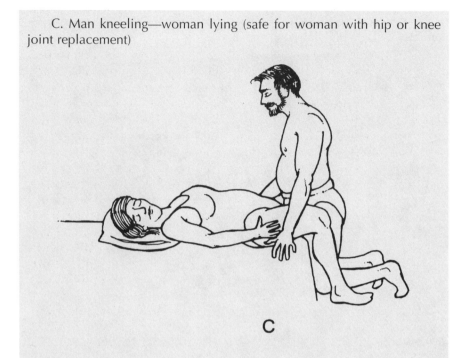

C

D. Side-lying (safe for man or woman with joint replacement. Operated extremity should lie on bottom)

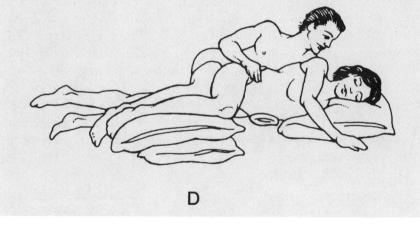

D

FIGURE 4-4   (continued)

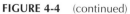

CASE REPORT—THE HIP

Tim and Audrey were understandably excited with the birth of their first child, a girl they named Gail. Gail weighed 6 pounds 7 ounces at birth and was otherwise healthy. Because Audrey had a family history of congenital dislocation of the hip, her obstetrician and pediatrician were alerted to this possibility. Examination in the newborn nursery disclosed an unstable left hip. This was confirmed by an ultrasound examination. An appropriate splint was applied that maintained the femoral head in its socket. However, subsequent X-rays as Gail grew failed to show normal development of the acetabulum despite the fact that she wore her brace day and night except for bathing. An arthrogram (an X-ray taken with absorbable dye injected into the joint) revealed that a marked infolding of soft tissue was preventing the femoral head from entering the acetabulum. An operation to correct this was performed, and the head was concentrically reduced into its socket. There were no complications such as collapse of the articular cartilage. Splinting was maintained for a long period after surgery, and the hip has developed normally. It was unnecessary to consider an operation either to build a bony shelf over the socket or to realign the acetabulum so as to contain the head.

QUESTIONS AND ANSWERS—THE HIP

Q: Do tumors occur in the hip as well as in other joints?

A: Both benign and malignant tumors can occur in and about the joints. These tumors (neoplasms: Gr. neo = new, plasm = formation) can arise from bone, cartilage, fibrous soft tissue, or vascular structures in or about the joint. Diagnosis is made with imaging (X-ray, CT scan, MRI, ultrasound), blood tests, and biopsy. Treatment usually is local excision for a benign growth. More aggressive surgery, including limb-salvage procedures, in which an entire joint may be removed and replaced with a bone graft and/or prosthesis, are available for malignant tumors. Radiation therapy and chemotherapy are sometimes indicated.

Q: What is heterotopic ossification?

A: Heterotopic ossification is a condition in which soft tissues (usually muscle) undergo changes in which they turn to bone. It can be caused by injury with bleeding into muscles around a joint. It has been seen after joint surgery. In its extreme form, it presents as a disease called *myositis ossificans* (muscle-inflammation-bone-formation), in which many muscles turn to bone. In the case of a single joint, excision of the bony mass after it matures can free the joint, although recurrence is not uncommon. There are medicines that prevent ossification as well as antiinflammatory drugs that can be taken prophylactically.

Q: What is bone cement?

A: Bone cement is polymethyl methacrylate, which comes as a powder and liquid that are mixed at the operating table, where it takes on a putty-like consistency, setting within a few minutes to provide rigid fixation of a prosthetic component. Although used in dentistry and some of the other surgical specialties for many years, it was first used to fix the components of a total hip by the English orthopaedic surgeon, Sir John Charnley, toward the middle of the twentieth century. This technique provided a quantum leap in the orthopaedic management of joint disease.

Q: What is proximal femoral focal deficiency?

A: Proximal femoral focal deficiency is a congenital abnormality of the proximal (near) part of the femur (thigh bone) and hip joint. Because of absence of the hip, the infant has a markedly shortened leg that does not grow along with the rest of his body. To date, there is no way to replace the missing hip joint. Treatment involves operations to the shortened leg so that an appropriate prosthesis can be fitted.

Q: Can congenital dislocation of the hip be diagnosed in a newborn infant?

A: A careful examination by an experienced observer can make the diagnosis of congenital dislocation of the hip at birth. This includes a variety of tests that reveal the hip to be unstable. It is important to make a diagnosis of congenital dislocation of the hip because the earlier treatment is started the easier it is to reduce and hold the hip in place so it will develop normally.

Q: Are there treatments for aseptic necrosis of the hip?

A: Aseptic necrosis of the hip is a serious condition that leads to collapse and irregularity of the articular surface of the femoral head. Early treatment includes relieving the hip from weight bearing using a brace and/or crutches. Because aseptic necrosis is due to a disruption of blood supply, surgical procedures to improve circulation such as removing dead bone and/or grafting new bone into the femoral head and neck sometimes are successful.

Now that we have had a look at the deepest joint in the body, let's visit the largest joint, its next-door neighbor, the knee.

5

The Knee

The knee is the largest of the 187 joints in the body (the smallest are those of the three ossicles of the inner ear). As such, the knee is subject to a variety of diseases and is frequently injured because it is commonly abused. The human knee was not designed to withstand the excessive strain that is often placed on it, particularly by weekend athletes.

Damage to knee ligaments is the most common ski injury, and knee ligament injuries occur more frequently in recreational basketball players than all other injuries combined. More people visit orthopaedic surgeons for problems with their knees than with any other complaint. Almost half a million knee operations are performed yearly in the United States. Nearly 70 percent of all football players will have knee surgery by the time they are in their mid-20s.

How do you know when you have a knee problem?—when it is painful, when it is swollen, because of either soft tissue swelling about the knee or an accumulation of fluid or blood within the knee. An easy way to see if your knee is inflamed is to place your hand on the front of your thigh and then place the same hand over the unaffected knee, which should feel cooler than the thigh. If the injured knee is as warm or warmer than the thigh, chances are it is inflamed. You also can feel how much warmer the swollen knee is than the unaffected one. Another sign of knee impairment is stiffness, which is nature's way of splinting a damaged joint; or locking (when it cannot be moved at all); or when it gives way on weight bearing. These signs or symptoms can be acute (sudden) or chronic (longstanding).

Walking up stairs places at least three times your body weight on the knee at each step, and walking down stairs subjects the knee (as well as the hip) to more than seven times your weight! That is why the cartilage that covers the knee must be thicker than anywhere else in the body. The knee is very vulnerable to sprains or strains. Arthritis, both degenerative and inflammatory, can affect the knee.

ANATOMY

The knee is a hinged joint with some rotation to provide locking. Two cartilage pads separate the knee bones. These are called the semilunar cartilages or menisci (Greek: meniskos = a crescent moon). Their purpose is to widen the articular surface and provide cushioning and shock absorption. These cartilages are frequently injured, especially the inside (medial) one. This usually occurs in sports that require cutting and twisting, such as football or soccer.

Four major ligaments stabilize the knee. The two *collateral* ligaments bind the femur to the tibia medially and laterally (inside and outside), and the two *cruciate* ligaments (which cross inside the joint) prevent the knee from unduly slipping forward or backward. A large pad of fat fills the space just below the patella (Figure 5-1).

INJURY

Knee ligaments, especially the medial collateral and anterior (front) cruciate ligaments, are prone to stretching and tearing with injury. An example of this is breaststroker's knee, a stress injury to the inside of the knee that is incurred during the breaststroke kick and is found in competitive swimmers. In violent injuries, such as those sustained in sports such as football or rugby, it is not uncommon to have tears of the medial meniscus associated with rupture of both the medial collateral and anterior cruciate ligaments—this is called the "terrible triad."

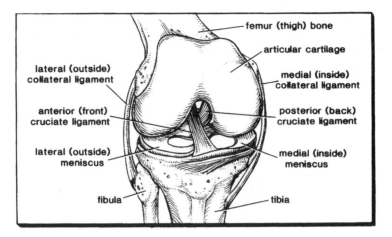

FIGURE 5-1 Your knee anatomy.

Most knee injuries are treated with arthroscopic techniques, both for diagnosis and for therapy. The word *arthroscopy* comes from two Greek words "arthro" (joint) and "skopein" (to look). In the examination the surgeon makes a small incision in the patient's skin and inserts a thin arthroscope, a tube about the diameter of a pencil and containing a miniature lens and lighting system that illuminates and magnifies the structures in the joint. Light is transmitted through fiberoptic cables using a small television camera and monitor combination, enabling the surgeon to see the interior of the joint, determine what is wrong, and perform a variety of surgical procedures. Such operations include repair or removal of a torn meniscus; repair or reconstruction of a ligament such as the anterior cruciate; shaving of an irregular, roughened patella or smoothing of other uneven surfaces; abrasion of bone with a burr to stimulate growth of fibrocartilage; removal of a thickened synovial lining and/or cartilaginous or bony loose bodies from the knee; or placing a meniscal implant, in which a damaged cartilage is replaced with a donor meniscus or an artificial substitute.

RECONSTRUCTIVE SURGERY

Reconstructive procedures for the damaged or degenerated knee include:

❑ *Autologous (from the patient) cartilage cell implantation.* This allows surgeons to harvest cells from a patient's own cartilage; the cells subsequently are cultured and then implanted into the knee to repair and resurface areas of cartilage loss.

❑ *Osteochondral autograft.* A technique somewhat like a hair-plug transfer, in which surgeons remove small sections of the patient's own bone and cartilage from an area of the knee that does not bear weight, transferring these plugs to a damaged portion of the knee.

❑ *Allograft reconstruction.* When there is a large area of bone and cartilage loss, the surgeon can implant a piece of freshly donated cartilage and bone that eventually functions as if it were the patient's own tissue.

Some of these procedures cannot be accomplished entirely through an arthroscope but require additional incisions for full visualization and instrumentation.

MUSCLE STRENGTH

The large muscles of the thigh provide strength and stability to the knee, particularly the quadriceps muscle group in the front and the hamstrings in the back. The quadriceps have four (L. quadri-) heads (L. caput) or parts. The five muscles whose tendons are severed when an animal is "hamstrung" in order to cripple it are called (you guessed it!) the hamstrings. Both these muscle groups weaken and waste rapidly after knee injury. Maintaining muscle tone is important in preventing injury as well as in rehabilitation after injury or surgery.

Disuse atrophy (wasting) caused by immobilization of the knee, for whatever reason, can delay recovery. It is the inside portion of the quadriceps that allows people to attain the upright posture. Apes walk in a crouched posture because they lack this muscle. It is the first muscle to waste after injury, making it difficult to walk upright. For this reason, exercising is very important to maintain healthy knees. Some exercises, however, particularly full knee squats, place a great deal of strain on the cruciate ligaments and should be avoided. The maximum force across the knee occurs at 35° of flexion. This means that

A. *Step-ups.* Find an object such as a large book that will support your weight. Step onto it until your leg is straight. Step down and repeat. As your knee gains strength you can increase the height of the step.

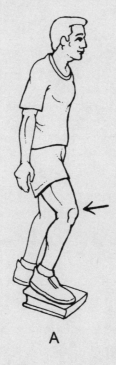

A

B. *Quadriceps setting or tightening.* Lie with knee extended. Tighten thigh muscles by pushing back of knee to the floor, making the leg as stiff as possible. Hold position for slow count of 6. Relax, then repeat.

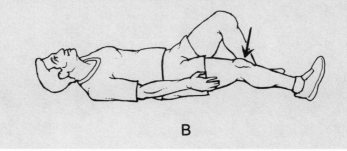

B

FIGURE 5-2   Exercises for rehabilitation of the knee.

C. *Leg bending.* Lie on stomach with both legs straight. Bend knee back as much as you can. Hold for a slow count of 6, then let foot down slowly. Rest and repeat.

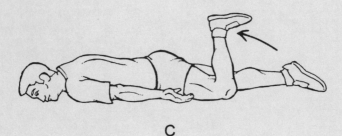

C

D. *Wall slides.* Stand with feet 12–18 inches from wall and lean back. Keep back flat against wall with legs straight. Slowly slide down wall until knees are slightly bent. Slowly push back up wall until knees are straight. Add an extra wall slide a day until you can perform 10–15 comfortably.

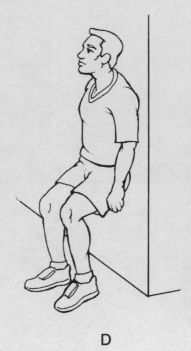

D

FIGURE 5-2   (continued)

E. *Leg lifts.* Comfortably seated, with knees bent, as illustrated, slowly lift your foot to the front until knee is straight, then press it under you as far as possible. Rest and repeat 10–12 times.

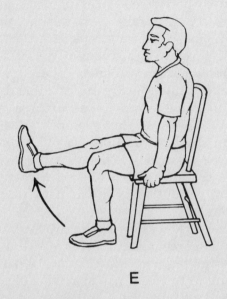

E

All of these exercises should be performed slowly. Start with 2–5 repetitions and work up to 25–30 as tolerated.

FIGURE 5-2   (continued)

more than seven times body weight is being transmitted to the knee during a deep knee bend. It is better to use isometric exercises (which involve contraction of the muscles without moving the knee, see page 49), isotonic exercise (in which a relatively constant level of tension is mainatained while moving the knee), isokinetic exercises (resistance exercising performed with the aid of a machine), range of motion exercises, stretching, biking, swimming, and aerobics as tolerated.

DIAGNOSIS

The diagnosis of a knee disorder is similar to the diagnosis of a problem in any other joint. A history will be taken, in particular asking about any injury, and a physical examination will be conducted. Aspiration of a swollen knee with analysis of the fluid obtained for cells and crystals such as those found in gout or pseudogout may be performed. Imaging, such as X-ray, CT, or MRI, will be ordered. X-rays taken with the knee under stress may be necessary to diagnose instability related to ligament laxity.

Diagnostic arthroscopy is frequently used in the management of knee problems. Many famous knees have been arthroscoped. Such superathletes as gymnast Mary Lou Retton and marathoner Joan Benoit underwent arthroscopy just before qualifying for the 1984 Olympic games. The ballet dancer Mikhail Baryshnikov had his knee looked into twice! General anesthesia may be required, although arthroscopy can be performed with a local anesthetic. Most arthroscopic procedures are done on an outpatient basis and do not require an overnight stay in the hospital.

Although knee arthroscopy in the proper hands is diagnostically close to 100 percent accurate, it is still a surgical procedure and has a complication rate of up to 15 percent, including damage to articular cartilage, postoperative bleeding, and even instrument breakage in the joint during the procedure. Recovery after knee surgery includes cautious weight bearing. The temporary use of crutches or a cane may be required. Rest with ice packs initially and rehabilitation exercises are prescribed, and a cast or brace sometimes may be necessary.

PATHOLOGY

Bursitis

The knee is surrounded by a number of bursae that may become inflamed and swollen. A common bursitis at the knee is housemaid's knee, which occurs in the bursal sac that lies just in front of the patella (kneecap). This occurred frequently in the pre–Minute-Maid mop era when housemaids knelt on their knees while scrubbing floors.

Bursitis of the infra- (below) patellar bursa occurs in coal miners who kneel while removing coal from narrow seams. Yet another bursitis at the back of the knee is called a Baker's cyst (after the man who first described it, not the trade).

Trauma

The automobile was the source of some unusual diseases in the early twentieth century, when it was considered an exotic means of transportation. One of these was chauffeur's knee, a partial ankylosis (stiffening) of the right knee caused by bracing the body to repeatedly turn the engine crank.

Like any joint, the knee can be fractured, ligaments can be torn, and the knee joint may even dislocate with severe force. For instance, contrary to what many people believe, water skiing can be a dangerous sport. Water is noncompressible, and the leverage exerted by the skis during a high-speed fall can cause severe damage to the knees.

Deformity

Various deformities of the knees are seen in children. Knock-knee and bowleg usually are self-limited but may persist into adolescence and may require surgical correction. Bony infection (osteomyelitis) and malignant bone tumor (osteogenic sarcoma) develop more often about the knee than at any other site. This is due to the rapid rate of growth of the bones at the knee.

Knee pain in a child may be due to a variety of conditions. Some of the more common are:

Osgood-Schlatter disease, immortalizing the two physicians who first diagnosed the condition—This is an inflammation at the insertion of the tendon of the patella (kneecap) onto the upper end of the tibia (large lower leg bone). It is an overuse syndrome most frequently found during puberty in boys, who stress their knees more often than girls. It is treated by rest and wearing a padded knee guard (occasionally a protective plaster cast). The condition is self-limited, but the patient may be left with a bump in front of his knee, which is no problem unless he enters a profession that requires frequent kneeling, such as the priesthood.

Stress fracture of the tibia—This is due to repetitive injury. Treatment is with rest and support.

Osteochondritis dissecans—This is a local avascular necrosis within the knee, with separation of a free fragment of bone and its overlying cartilage. It usually is managed with rest. Operative fixation of the free fragment is required if it is large, loose, or displaced.

Meniscal lesions or injury—The usual meniscus is semilunar in shape. When a meniscus is shaped like a disk, it can cause snapping, limited range of motion, and sometimes locking and pain in the knee. MRI and arthroscopic examination may be necessary to confirm the diagnosis. Complete excision should be avoided. Surgery to reshape the meniscus is available.

A torn meniscus often can be repaired to maintain normal knee function. A variety of tools are available for such a procedure, including bioabsorbable sutures and staples as well as metal darts or screws. Sometimes a meniscus is so severely damaged that it must be completely removed. This operation can decrease the shock-absorbing capacity of the knee by as much as 20 percent and can lead to a cascade of events in which the knee degenerates and eventually becomes arthritic. One option for slowing this degeneration is meniscal allograft (tissue banked human graft) transplantation.

Chondromalacia patellae—This is the most common patellar disorder. It is an overuse syndrome with onset during adolescence. Chondromalacia patellae is frequently seen in teenagers during rapid spurts of growth. It is more common in girls and could be related to hormonal change during adolescence. Patients experience crepitation (grinding) on knee motion and pain after prolonged sitting with the knees bent. Softening and shredding of the articular cartilage of the patella occurs. Management includes appropriate exercises, rest, elastic knee supports, and nonsteroidal antiinflammatory drugs. Occasionally, surgery with smoothing of the roughened patella is indicated.

Patellar subluxation (slipping) or dislocation (slipped)—This can occur in the dysplastic (poorly formed) lax knee. Treatment may include the use of an elastic or neoprene knee sleeve support to help keep the patella from slipping (usually to the outside of the knee). Exercises to strengthen the muscles holding the patella in place sometimes will help. The patella may be realigned within the femoral groove by any of a number of operations that either release the tight muscle on the outside of the knee that causes the patella to slip to the side; by tightening the muscle on the inside of the knee, which holds the patella in place; or by transferring the insertion of the patellar tendon to enable the patella to track more normally during movements of the knee.

Popliteal (fossa in the back of the knee) or Baker's cysts—These are synovial swellings that usually resolve in a year or two and require only observation. Excision is indicated for large, painful, or persistent cysts or when the diagnosis is uncertain.

ARTHRITIS

The knee is frequently the site of arthritis. Osteoarthritis causes loss of the cartilage "cushion" of the knee. As this wears away, bones become rough and rub together, causing pain. Arthroscopic debridement (removal of loose pieces of bone, cartilage, and soft tissue through an arthroscope) can provide relief. Lavage (flushing) of the joint with large amounts of sterile fluid can help wash out tissue fragments and crystals and dilute enzymes that are part of the degradative process of osteoarthritis. Viscosupplementation (injection of a substance that offers relief from pain by lubricating the joint) is another cutting edge therapy. Osteotomy sometimes can provide relief. This is a procedure in which the thigh or shin bone is cut to realign the leg, shifting the weight-bearing burden from the painful portion of the knee, where cartilage is missing or damaged, to a healthier, stronger portion of the knee.

Finally, a *unicompartmental* (either the medial or lateral compartment only) arthroplasty of the knee that involves resurfacing only one damaged side of the knee, or a total knee replacement for more extensive arthritis, can be performed. There are a variety of total knee replacements that can be customized to any particular anatomy or pathology. State-of-the-art technology includes "mobile-bearing" implants that rotate and pivot as the knee moves, permitting optimal congruency and resulting in less wear. Orthopaedic surgeons who specialize in total joint replacement not infrequently replace both knees at the same time when indicated. The operation involves removing diseased and damaged tissue, reshaping the bones, inserting the prosthesis, and sometimes reconstructing the ligaments of the joint. It often is desirable to donate your own blood before your hospital stay because you may need blood transfusions during the surgery. Early motion is provided through an exercise machine that moves your leg (a continuous passive motion machine). Early walking is encouraged, with strengthening exercises, a walker, and assistance. Blood thinners are often given to avoid the problem of blood clots after surgery.

Allograft knees have been transplanted in younger patients in whom there is complete loss of the joint and its supporting tissues. Such patients require immunosuppressive drugs for life to avoid rejection of the foreign graft tissue, but otherwise they fare well.

CASE REPORT—THE KNEE

Shirley R. was a 16-year-old high school cheerleader who began to experience pain in her right knee. This was particularly severe when bending the knees or just after getting up from a chair and climbing stairs. Shirley tried applying heat to her knees and taking some over-the-counter medications. This provided insignificant relief. She was seen by her family physician, who referred her to an orthopaedic surgeon.

Examination revealed that Shirley had mild knock-knee and that the undersurface of the medial side of the right patella was tender to pressure. An X-ray of the knee was negative except for a special "sky line" view, which showed that the groove in which the kneecap slides was shallow on one side. Some mild crepitation (grinding) was felt on moving the patella. A diagnosis of an overuse syndrome, chondromalacia patellae, was made, and Shirley was instructed in isometric quadriceps strengthening exercises and cautioned to curtail her activities, particularly avoiding those that created pain. Vitamin C and aspirin were prescribed. She was given a neoprene knee sleeve for patellar support.

Most cases of modest chondromalacia patellae are self-limited and usually resolve by the end of adolescence. If Shirley does not improve with time or if her knees become worse, an arthroscopic shaving of the irregular surface of her patella may be necessary.

QUESTIONS AND ANSWERS—THE KNEE

> **Q:** How is it possible for the knee (and the hip) to bear three times body weight at each step when ascending stairs and up to more than seven times body weight when walking down stairs?
>
> **A:** Your body weight of course doesn't change. However, the force at weight-bearing impact coupled with the compressive force generated in the muscles that stabilize the knee and hip subject these joints to markedly increased load during stair-walking.

Q: What accounts for the excruciating pain that sometimes occurs with even a minor knee injury?

A: The synovial membranes and fat pads are very rich in sensory nerve fibers. This accounts for the sickening pain that accompanies any injury to the joint.

Q: What is the difference between fibrocartilage and hyaline cartilage?

A: Fibrocartilage is a thick collagen substance much like fibrous tissue elsewhere in the body. Hyaline cartilage is the special articular cartilage found lining joints. When hyaline cartilage wears out, the supporting bone underneath can be surgically abraded or drilled. This initiates a healing response that forms fibrocartilage (not hyaline cartilage), which fills in the eroded areas in the joint.

Q: Are pain fibers the only nerves serving joints?

A: Sensory fibers from the joint capsule are of two kinds: *pain fibers*, which are stimulated when the capsule or other ligaments are overstretched or torn; and *proprioceptive fibers*, which convey information regarding the position of the joint at rest and when in motion. Repeated injury to the joint decreases this proprioceptive ability, leading to joint instability with further damage.

Q: Is knee fusion (arthrodesis) a serious operation?

A: Very serious indeed. It is a "court of last resort" for the painful, completely degenerated, and/or unstable knee. Although ministering angels have no knees because they must always stand in the presence of God, we humans require a movable knee to function well as mobile creatures. Although it is still possible to get around, work, and even engage in modest athletic activity with one stiff knee, it can be difficult to drive an automobile and it is almost impossible to ride a bicycle. Among other annoyances, you will always have to sit in an aisle seat at a theater.

Q: Who has more knee injuries, men or women?

A: The anatomic characteristics of the female body make a woman's knees more vulnerable to injury. This is because their hips are wider, which causes the thigh bones to turn inward, putting more pressure on the knees. The extra width of the hips also contributes to knock-knee.

Finally, women have 20 percent less muscle mass then men. So, pound for pound, there is less muscle to support the knee.

Q: What are pathologic synovial plicae?

A: These are the thin membranous walls that separated the three knee compartments during embryonic development. As developmental leftovers, they are found in up to 50 percent of normal knees. These bands, like postsurgical adhesions in the abdomen, sometimes can cause acute or chronic knee pain. Arthroscopic release or removal of an annoying plica is sometimes required.

Q: Is it necessary to remove the entire meniscus when only part of a meniscus is torn?

A: It is not only unnecessary but also undesirable because the meniscus protects the knee from developing osteoarthritis. Well over 90 percent of the 100,000 or so meniscectomies performed yearly in the United States are only partial. Additionally, if the tear is along the margin of the meniscus where blood supply is adequate, it often can be sewn up and will heal.

Q: What is the Cybex machine that is used at some sports medicine centers?

A: The Cybex machine matches a patient's resistance during exercise. The apparatus can measure range of motion, power, strength, and endurance. These capabilities are recorded by a computer, and the resulting printout is used to keep track of a patient's rehabilitation. The Cybex also can reveal otherwise unrecognized muscle weakness. Thus, a customized muscle strengthening program can be prescribed.

Q: Is it always necessary to repair torn ligaments in the knee?

A: Immobilizing the knee in an appropriate cast or brace often will allow a torn collateral ligament to heal as well as if it had been repaired surgically. In the case of the anterior cruciate ligament, its absence can leave very little instability or functional disability for the person who does not stress his or her knees. A strong quadriceps muscle often can compensate for a torn anterior cruciate, and, except in cases of professional athletes who require

"Cadillac" knees, the absence of this ligament does not preclude participation in modest recreational athletics.

The professional athlete or even the serious amateur (particularly those engaged in sports that require cutting and twisting) is, of course, a different problem. But repair of the ligament can be difficult and must be supplemented with other natural tissue such as a slip from the patellar tendon or an artificial ligament made of a carbon composite. Rehabilitation may be prolonged and involved, requiring a brace and often taking as long as a year. Reconstruction of a torn anterior cruciate ligament is not a procedure to be taken lightly.

Q: What rehabilitation is required after knee surgery?

A: Surgery without rehabilitation is useless. Rehabilitation involves specific exercises, starting with quadriceps drill without weights and progressing to weights as tolerated.

Even without surgery, braces are used to provide immobility and facilitate soft tissue repair, and exercises are prescribed to stimulate muscle strengthening. Rehabilitation is programmed into three phases: (1) a phase of rest, (2) a phase of exercise to rebuild strength and endurance, and (3) a phase of conditioning for full functional performance.

Special rehabilitative techniques include water workouts that involve exercising in a pool to take advantage of both the buoyancy provided to an injured limb and the resistance afforded by the water. Range of motion exercises are used to help regain full joint movement; strengthening exercises increase power; functional exercises recover useful movements; stretching exercises stretch out contractures; and aerobic exercise increases flexibility and endurance.

Q: Which meniscus is more frequently torn?

A: The inside (medial) meniscus is more frequently torn because it is larger, more mobile, and more vulnerable. The outer (lateral) meniscus can also be torn. Wrestlers are more likely to suffer lateral tears.

Healing is very poor because more than 70 percent of the meniscus is without a blood supply. The only meniscal tears that lend themselves to repair rather than excision are those at the outer margin, where the blood supply is more plentiful. Incidentally, once a meniscus is removed, nothing like the original cartilage will grow back in its place.

Q: What is the Lenox Hill brace?

A: This is a custom-made appliance that was popularized in 1969 by the New York Jets quarterback Joe Namath. It is a derotation appliance that weighs less than two pounds and has seven straps supporting the knee externally in the same way it would normally be supported internally by intact ligaments. The brace may cost as much as $1,000, but it is well worth it if you need one.

Q: Is it possible to function without your kneecap?

A: Some people must have the kneecap removed because it is shattered or severely arthritic. The knee cannot then function normally, but you can get by reasonably well without a kneecap. The kneecap acts as a pulley for quadriceps muscle action, and in its absence the quadriceps tendon falls back onto the joint as it contracts to straighten the knee. The muscle must be at least 30 percent stronger in order to stabilize the knee as well as it did before removal of the kneecap.

Q: What causes knock-knee and bowlegs?

A: Genu valgum (knock-knee) and genu varum (bowlegs) can be present in normal children during early growth. Both "deformities" often are carryovers from the tight-packed intrauterine position of the fetus. Rickets (lack of vitamin D with subsequent abnormality of bony calcification) can cause knee deformities including bowing. Other pathologic causes include damage to the growth plate, infection, arthritis, osteochondral dysplasia (bone-cartilage-abnormality of growth), and Blount's disease, which is a growth disorder of the inner portion of the tibial growth plate that produces a localized varus deformity and bowlegs. Appropriate treatment, including bracing and surgery, is available for each of these conditions.

Q: Which total joint replacement was developed first—the hip or the knee?

A: As we read in the last chapter, the earliest total hip replacement was documented in 1891 by the German surgeon Theophilus Gluck. In 1860 Verneuil interposed soft tissue between the bones of the temporomandibular joint, and in 1863 this technique was applied to the knee. Subsequently, nylon, muscle, fat, cellophane, fascia, and pig bladder were used as interpositional resurfacing materials. In 1940 Willis Campbell reported one of the earliest uses of metal in knee arthroplasty, and in 1958 MacIntosh described an acrylic tibial prosthesis (later modified to chrome-cobalt) inserted in the arthritic knee to correct deformity, restore stability, and relieve pain.

Continuing our skeletal journey, let's now drop down and visit the ankle.

6

The Ankle

"The innocent ankle and blameless instep are tortured
for the vices of the nobler organs."
Sidney Smith Letter (on gout) to the Countess of Carlisle
September 5, 1840

ANATOMY

The *tibia* (shin bone) and *fibula* (thin outside bone of the leg, Latin = needle) embrace the *talus* bone of the foot to form the ankle joint. Talus means die, because sheep tali are square and were used as dice for games in the ancient Middle East. Roman soldiers used such sheep tali to gamble for Christ's clothes at the time of his crucifixion.

In its weight-bearing position, stability of the ankle joint is favored by the congruence of its articular surface, ligamentous support, and associated muscle activity. The ankle is firmest in the close-packed position of dorsiflexion (bent upward) and is most vulnerable to torque stress in the loose-packed position of plantar flexion (bent downward). The ligamentous structures along the medial (inside) of the joint provide more stability than do the lateral (outside) ligaments. For these reasons, injury to the joint most often occurs when it is being twisted down and in. Movement at the ankle is supplemented by motion between the talus and the calcaneus (heel bone) of the foot (Figure 6-1).

Injury to the Ankle

The ankle has been increasingly subjected to stress and trauma because of the popularization of physical activities, particularly

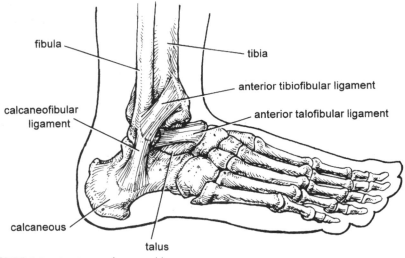

FIGURE 6-1 Anatomy of your ankle.

competitive athletics. The major predisposing factors for injury are inadequate training resulting in overuse of the joint and improper equipment, particularly footwear. However, not everyone is biomechanically perfect even with adequate training, and this, in conjunction with the force of superincumbent body weight, can create problems. The following conditions most commonly affect the ankle.

LATERAL LIGAMENT SPRAIN   Sprain of the lateral ligament of the ankle is the most common injury that occurs in sports. The trauma usually is sustained when landing on a foot that is plantar flexed (bent downward) and inverted (twisted in) from a jump, or when running. In this position, the lateral ligament is subjected to the greatest stress and is likely to tear. Once torn, the ankle is rendered unstable. Swelling, tenderness, bruising, and pain with loss of range of motion are present. There is difficulty in weight bearing because of pain. X-rays fail to reveal a fracture.

If the sprain is minimal, with tearing of only a few fibers, it can be treated with Rest, Ice, Compression (the foot should be wrapped tighter than the ankle with an elastic bandage so that swelling is squeezed out toward the heart), and Elevation (R-I-C-E) for the first 24 to 72 hours. Early mobility exercises and isometric strengthening are prescribed as tolerated. An engaging exercise for maintaining ankle range of motion is to trace the alphabet from A to Z in the air, moving the foot at the ankle. Weight bearing is encouraged, with or without crutches in accordance with the presence or absence of pain. An elastic or neoprene ankle support or an air brace, which braces the ankle stirrup-fashion with inflated padding, is sometimes advised. Proprioceptive exercises (using a wobble-board) are desirable after healing has occurred because repeat injuries can damage proprioception (position sense) in the ankle.

When the sprain is more severe and results in complete ligamentous disruption, a plaster cast for older people and primary surgical repair for the younger athlete is the treatment of choice. A plaster cast is worn for approximately 10 days after surgical repair, followed by the application of a functional splint for six weeks. Similar diagnostic criteria and the same treatment format apply for ligamentous injuries to the medial aspect of the joint.

FRACTURES   Any type of fracture can occur in the ankle joint, depending on the mechanism and severity of the force applied. The injury usually is twisting in nature, or the trauma may involve compression such as that incurred in a fall from a height. Shear or torqued stresses can rupture ligaments and fracture bones.

Fractures are classified according to the mechanism of injury, the bones fractured, the ligaments torn, and the displacement of fracture fragments. Uncomplicated fractures often can be managed by closed *reduction* (manipulative correction) of the fracture (which may require a general anesthetic for muscle relaxation) and application of a plaster cast for an appropriate length of time to hold the bone fragments in place until healing occurs. More complicated fractures may require surgery with reduction and fixation with pins, screws, staples, and/or metal plates. After surgery, a cast may be necessary for a brief period of time, but usually not as long as when the treatment is closed (nonsurgical).

Current technology offers absorbable (also called bioabsorbable or resorbable) fixation devices. These are screws, pins, staples, and plates made of compounds that can be absorbed over time by the patient's body. Such devices are claimed to be safer than the metal devices traditionally used in orthopaedic surgery. Unlike absorbable devices, metal fixation devices sometimes must be removed, and this requires a second surgical procedure. They also can become colonization sites for bacteria, leading to infection. The most popular use for absorbable fixation devices today is attaching ligaments and tendons to bone and repairing torn menisci in the knee.

OTHER ANKLE DISORDERS   *Osteochondritis dissecans* can occur in the ankle (the bone involved usually is the talus), where it is treated like the similar condition occurring in the knee.

Although osteoarthritis of the ankle is unusual, it may happen secondary to an ankle fracture. Arthritis can develop following a displaced ankle fracture if the joint has not been returned to its normal anatomy. Secondary degeneration will be evident on X-ray some months following the injury. Indications for surgery are a painful ankle that is not improving at least 18 months after fracture. Operations include arthrodesis (fusion) of the ankle by one of a variety of methods or replacement of the diseased bone with a plastic and metal prosthesis. The surgical decision is made on the basis of the patient's age and lifestyle, as well as the skill and experience of the surgeon. Total ankle replacement has not, by and large, been as successful a procedure as total replacement of the hip or knee.

RUNNING INJURY   Runners with excessively mobile ankles unduly flatten their feet while running. This may cause lateral ankle pain. A runner usually reports that his ankle "gives out." The problem may have existed during childhood but usually becomes significant only when the athlete begins long-distance training. This can be treated by an appropriate wedge in the running shoe or a rigid heel counter and reinforced shoe upper to correct the flat foot. Isometric exercises to strengthen the muscles in the outside compartment of the leg can be performed by pushing the foot out against an immovable object while seated with the knee bent and the ankle held at a right angle (90°) with the foot.

Both horses and humans have evolved a lengthy, efficient stride by developing legs that are long relative to the body. In the horse the foot has lengthened, placing the heel (hock) high above the ground. In humans the thigh and shin segments of the leg have elongated. Through its complex of leg joints the horse can sprint at the gallop to nearly 70 kilometers per hour—almost twice the speed of human athletes. Even though we humans lack

---

CASE REPORT—THE ANKLE

Howard T. was a 26-year-old "weekend warrior." During the week he worked as a stockbroker. On the weekend Howard liked to run and scrimmage at basketball with friends at his local YMCA. He used a pair of well-worn running shoes for both activities. One Sunday morning, while coming down from an attempted slam dunk, Howard landed on the outside of his right foot, violently twisting the foot in at the ankle. He collapsed on the spot because his foot and ankle could no longer bear his weight. There was immediate severe pain with swelling along the outside of the ankle. Howard was taken home, where he elevated his ankle to relieve swelling, applied ice, and asked his wife to go to the drugstore to purchase an elastic bandage, which he applied. He had difficulty sleeping that night as a result of the pain. The next morning he went to see his doctor and was referred to an orthopaedic surgeon.

By this time the area of injury was black and blue because of bleeding from soft tissue tearing. Although an X-ray failed to show a fracture, a stress X-ray, which is taken while the ankle is stretched, revealed abnormal laxity of the outside aspect of the joint. A diagnosis of rupture of the lateral ligament was made, a plaster splint was applied, and crutch-walking was advised for comfort. Because of Howard's age and his desire to continue athletics, surgical repair of the torn ligament was advised. Severe soft tissue disruption was noted at surgery. The torn ligament was matched end-to-end and securely sewn back together. A plaster cast was worn for 10 days after surgery, and a functional plastic splint that could be removed for bathing and sleeping was worn for another six weeks. Howard engaged in intensive physical therapy, including strengthening exercises for his ankle. Approximately three months after surgery he gradually began to return to athletics wearing an elastic ankle support and appropriate athletic shoes with a high supportive shoe

---

the equine's complex biomechanics, we are still able to perform amazing feats of athletic skill because of the strength and agility of our hips, our knees, and, of course, our ankles.

QUESTIONS AND ANSWERS—THE ANKLE

Q: Although it is seldom involved in primary osteoarthritis, is the ankle ever involved in rheumatoid arthritis?

A: Yes, indeed. The ankle joint is a major weight-bearing joint and therefore one of the most frequently involved joints in rheumatoid arthritis. Treatment consists of medicines, rest, and appropriate support. Operations such as ankle replacement and ankle fusion are available for advanced cases.

Q: Is fusion of the ankle as disabling an operation as fusion of the knee?

A: Any surgical procedure that results in loss of joint movement can be disabling in and of itself. However, loss of motion at the ankle is not as serious as loss of motion at the knee. Ankle fusion has proven to be an excellent surgical salvage procedure to relieve pain and provide stability for standing and walking. Loss of ankle motion is to a degree compensated for by increased motion in the joints of the mid-portion of the foot. An important operative consideration in women is fusing the ankle in a position that will accommodate a high-heeled shoe.

Q: Can diabetes affect the ankle joint?

A: Diabetes can affect the nerves and blood vessels that serve joints. Position sense and sensation are lost, making the joint more vulnerable to injury. Disintegration of bones and cartilage can occur, resulting in a *neuropathic joint*. This occurs most frequently in the ankle and other weight-bearing joints. It is called a "Charcot joint" because it was first described by the great French neurologist Jean Martin Charcot (1825–1893).

Q: How are chronic ankle sprains treated?

A: Up to 20 percent of people who sprain an ankle will have some residual ankle weakness and functional instability, which may lead to recurrent ankle sprains. This chronic ankle sprain can be treated conservatively with physical therapy, including strengthening exercises, and bracing of the ankle. If the ankle does not improve, it can be treated surgically either by repairing torn ligaments or by transferring a nearby tendon to tighten the ankle by augmenting the strength of the ankle ligaments.

Now let's take a look at the last link in the chain that enables us to stand and move about—our feet.

7

The Foot

"Keep the head cool, the feet warm, and the bowels open."
Herman Boerhaave

Consider your feet! In an average day, they can absorb more than 700 tons of force. In your lifetime, by walking 1.2 x 106 steps each year, your feet carry you almost 75,000 miles, which is just about three times around the Earth's equator. The average man walks approximately six miles a day, the average woman nearly nine. While walking, an adult can exert almost 450 pounds of pressure on the feet with each step taken. It is small wonder, then, that foot problems reportedly affect nearly 43 million Americans and cost up to $3.5 billion annually.

Bipedal (two-footed) walking is seen only in primates and reaches its greatest sophistication in human beings. The process of developing our pattern of walking began several million years ago, freeing our arms and hands for creative tasks such as hunting, planting, and tool-making. Movement of the leg muscles assists the heart in pumping the blood. Prolonged inactivity, such as sitting on an airplane (particularly with the legs crossed), causes blood and other fluids to collect in the feet through gravity. You should avoid sitting for long periods, whether on a train, plane, bus, or even in an office. Get up and move around frequently so that your leg muscles have a chance to pump and keep your feet from swelling.

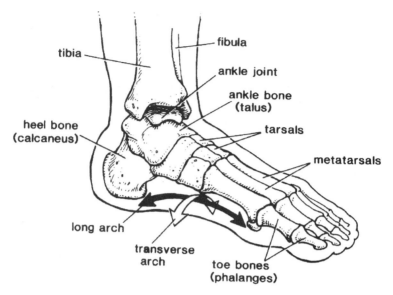

FIGURE 7-1   Anatomy of the foot.

STRUCTURE

Each foot has 26 bones that form two arches (Figure 7-1). The *transverse* (metatarsal) arch runs across the ball of the foot. Your *long* arch spans your instep. The arches function as shock absorbers and tend to flatten on weight bearing. Some people have *pes planus* (flatfoot). This usually is not a severe disability unless it is accompanied by spasticity of the peroneal muscles that lie on the outer side of the leg and serve the foot. Many great athletes have been flat-footed, and Native Americans, whose soft moccasins offered foot protection but minimal support, were habitually flat-footed. They were, however, able to climb, run, and track with amazing agility.

Until three or four years of age, children do not display a long arch because this area is filled with baby fat. Adolescent girls who have functional (postural) flatfeet will develop an arch when they begin wearing a higher heeled shoe. The only serious kind of flatfoot is the spastic type, which is accompanied by congenital fusion of several bones in the mid- or hind foot. Flattening of the long arch also may be due to a tight heel cord. Dropping of the transverse arch can occur secondary to conditions such as arthritis. High, rigid arches usually are more painful than flat arches and, in fact, may be indicative of a more generalized neuromuscular disorder.

The 33 joints of the foot keep it flexible. Foot movement is controlled by 38 muscles, originating both within and without the foot proper. The bones of the foot are held together by 56 ligaments, any of which may be strained or sprained during a twist or fall.

WALKING

A toddler first learning to walk tends to waddle, throwing his feet out (out-toeing). He does this to increase the width of his base of support to prevent falling. This condition as well as occasional pigeon-toeing (in-toeing) tend to resolve as the child gains balance with growth. Mild knock-knees or bowlegs are reflections of early incoordination and often are natural transitions as the infant "unwinds" from the curled position it had in the mother's womb. These "functional deformities" similarly resolve with growth.

Leonardo da Vinci claimed the feet to be "a masterpiece of engineering and a work of art." You must agree that your feet are amazing locomotor organs. Walking can best be described as a controlled fall. You lose balance, gain balance, lose balance, gain balance, over and over again. Your feet monitor rather than motivate ambulation. Most of the metabolic energy expended by the feet during walking is used to slow gait and keep the body from completely falling. To do this, each foot must make a step much like a jet airplane landing, with the wheels (heel) down and the nose (toes) up. Therefore, each step is a heel–toe rhythm with takeoff on your toes and full weight bearing on each foot alternately as the other swings through. On stance, weight is borne on the tripod of the heel, the base of the great toe, and the bottom of the fifth toe. Body weight is centered over the feet, the inner borders remaining rigid for support and the outer flexible to adapt to variations in the contour of the walking surface.

During walking the big toe maintains balance while the little toes work as a springboard. The outer two metatarsal bones move to adapt to uneven walking surfaces, while the three inner bones stay rigid for support. The long plantar ligament, one of the strongest ligaments in the body, helps the long arch maintain its resilience.

FOOTWEAR

The first human being stood upright about one million years ago, and people have suffered foot problems ever since. As II Chronicles, 16:12 notes, "... And Asa in the thirty and ninth year of his reign was diseased in his feet...." Today's high heels are rough on modern women's feet because they shift weight from the heels to the toes. Yet only 45 percent of American women acknowledge that they wear uncomfortable shoes because they look good. Men's feet have not fared too well either (20 percent of men admit to wearing shoes for looks, not comfort). Overeating and inactivity lead to obesity, and these extra pounds can make a pair of feet ache. Wearing improper footwear causes painful problems (it has been said that the cure for a headache is to wear tight shoes) and may contribute to thousands of hours of downtime at work. This translates into the loss of millions of dollars to industry each year.

Pads, bars, or heel cups are prescribed for feet that do not allow normal movement. These devices modify the shoe and are designed to assist motion by changing the way the bones, joints, and muscles work during ambulation.

Feet tend to spread in the forefoot under the burden of the body's weight and activity. This increases with age. Most shoes are designed to be more narrow in the forefoot than the foot itself, which can contribute to a variety of troublesome problems.

While standing with full weight on a piece of paper, trace around your foot. Now place your shoe directly over the tracing, and you can see if your forefoot is wider than your shoe. A proper shoe should accommodate the forefoot without pinching. The toe box should be rounded and roomy enough so you can wiggle all your toes, the heel should absorb shock, the sole should be skid-resistant, and the upper should be breathable.

WOMEN'S FEET

Foot pain and deformity is a particular problem for women. Even though foot size tends to increase after 20 years of age, most women have not had their feet measured in more than five years. As a result, women wear shoes that are too small.

This contributes to significant foot deformity and pain. As the foot gets longer, the width of the forefoot appears to increase, whereas heel width does not significantly change. Even though wearing stylish shoes may be painful, many women suffer for style, risking the development of deformities such as hammertoes and bunions. There are reasons severely styled shoes are less comfortable than well-fitted leisure shoes. Most shoe styles are copied from the Italian and French, whose feet are shaped differently than those of Americans. Most shoes manufactured abroad are available "narrow," "medium," or "wide" and are not specifically sized. Although the pointed toe originally was meant to be a false-front styling, a woman with a long foot, particularly if she wears a high-heeled shoe that slides the foot forward, ends up having her toes constricted by the tapered toe. To avoid painful constriction of the forefoot, women with long feet require a shoe with a "combination last," which has disproportionate forefoot and hind foot widths. However, shoes in numerous widths and styles are expensive to produce and stock, so manufacturers often cannot afford to make the combination last, and retailers hesitate to carry a large inventory.

Surveys show that adolescent girls tend to choose proper shoes (those with wide toe boxes and sufficient room) but that they make these choices for style, not comfort.

SELECTING SHOES

The following rules will ensure that you select shoes that fit properly:

1. Try on shoes at the end of the day, when your feet are largest. The toes should have room to move in an ample toe box. The end of the longest toe of the biggest foot should clear the end of the shoe by a finger's breadth. The foot should not bulge over the side of the shoe, and the upper should not wrinkle when the shoe is bent.
2. If possible, your shoes should be made of suede or soft leather. Synthetic materials and patent leather do not "give" when your foot changes shape as you walk.

3. Make sure that your shoes are comfortable when you buy them. Do not anticipate a "break-in" period for shoes.
4. The foot must not feel tight in the shoe, even though the counter should grip the heel snugly. Select the shoe by how it fits, not by the size of the shoe. Sizes vary by manufacturer.
5. When trying on shoes, always stand up and walk around in them.
6. When purchasing sports shoes, wear the socks you normally wear when you work out.
7. Sometimes differences between foot size and shoe fit can be corrected with shoe inserts. However, it is preferable to purchase shoes that fit correctly without modification.

The selection of proper athletic shoes sometimes presents a problem because people often select athletic shoes on the basis of design and color rather than fit. This can lead to foot strain and injury. A simple "footprint test" can help you select the appropriate shoe based on your foot type. Just wet your feet and stand on a sheet of newspaper. A normal print includes your heel, part of the midfoot, and the forefoot. This type of foot benefits from a stabilizing shoe that has a semicurved last. A flat foot will imprint the whole foot. Flat (pronated) feet require a shoe with a long arch support, a firm heel cup, and a straight

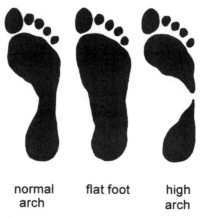

normal   flat foot   high
arch   arch

FIGURE 7-2   The footprint test.

last for motion control. A print showing only the forefoot and heel indicates a high-arched foot that is twisted in (supinated). Such feet are most comfortable in cushioned shoes built on a curved flexible last.

Soft tissue problems of the foot, including ingrown toenails, corns and calluses, plantar warts, athlete's foot, and the like, are covered in my book *All About Bone* (Demos, 1998). Some common problems involving the joints of the foot are as follows:

FRACTURES

Any bone in the foot may be broken, and fractures can involve any joint in the foot. Even when the fracture does not directly involve a joint, it may throw the joint out of alignment. Anatomic reduction is essential, and adequate immobilization with appropriate plaster casts or internal metallic fixation is necessary for restoration of painless foot function.

Fracture of the *calcaneus* (heel bone) is a serious injury that commonly results from a fall in which the patient lands on his heels. The long-term result following a displaced fracture is poor. The common sign of calcaneal injury is bruising on the instep of the foot. This is because the attachment of the plantar fascia limits the spread of bleeding. The injured heel may be wider than its uninjured mate. Tenderness in the thoracolumbar junction of the spine may be due to a vertebral crush fracture, which commonly accompanies a calcaneal injury. X-rays will confirm the diagnosis. Depending on the severity of the break, such fractures can often be treated by manipulation and casting. A calcaneal fracture with depression of the subtalar joint (between the talus and calcaneus) that is not comminuted (in many pieces) is suitable for elevation of the joint surface and internal fixation.

DIABETES

A special case is the diabetic foot, which requires close attention. Even mild diabetes eventually can cause damage to nerves and blood vessels, which in turn can lead to decreased sensation and circulation in the feet. Pressure sores, ulcers, and infection

CARE OF THE DIABETIC FOOT

1. Do not smoke.

2. Inspect toes and between toes daily for blisters, cuts, and scratches. Using a mirror can aid in seeing the bottom of the feet.

3. Wash feet daily and dry carefully, especially between toes.

4. Avoid extremes of temperatures. Test water by hand before bathing.

5. If feet feel cold at night, wear socks. Do not apply hot water bottles or heating pads.

6. Do not use chemical agents to remove corns an calluses.

7. Inspect inside of shoes daily for foreign objects, nail points, and torn linings.

8. Wear properly fitted stockings. Do not wear mended stockings. Avoid stockings with seams.

9. Do not wear garters.

10. Shoes should be comfortable at the time of purchase. Do not depend on them to stretch out.

11. Do not wear shoes without stockings.

12. Do not wear sandals with thongs between the toes.

13. Do not walk barefoot, especially on hot surfaces such as sandy beaches or around swimming pools.

14. Cut nails straight across.

15. Do not cut corns and calluses. Follow special instructions from your physician or podiatrist.

16. See your physician regularly and be sure that your feet are examined at each visit.

17. If your vision is impaired, have a family member inspect feet daily, trim nails, and buff down calluses.

18. Be sure to inform your podiatrist that you have diabetes.

result. Prevention is possible through close surveillance of the feet with daily inspection and immediate treatment of any scratches, abrasions, or pressure areas. Good foot hygiene is mandatory.

In the case of advanced diabetes, which may include damage to the bones and joints as well as the skin of the feet, hospitalization with bed rest, foot elevation, and intravenous administration of antibiotics becomes necessary. Casting of the foot and surgery to remove infected bone, as well as amputation in some cases, may be indicated.

HEEL PAIN

Heel pain is a common condition that can result from bursitis around the Achilles tendon as well as inflammation of the growth zone of the back of the heel bone (calcaneal apophysitis—Sever's disease) in a child.

Pain and tenderness at the point of the heel on weight bearing may be due to an inflammation of the plantar fascia (plantar fasciitis) as it originates from the weight-bearing portion of the os calcis (heel bone). A traction spur caused by pulling from the plantar fascia can occur at this point. Tightness of the Achilles tendon (heel cord) can contribute to the discomfort. This can be relieved by stretching exercises (see chart).

A. As illustrated, stand arm's length from wall, with one knee straight and the other bent. Supporting your body with your hands on the wall, lean forward toward the wall, keeping the knee straight and your heel flat on the floor. If done properly, you should feel your heel cord stretching.

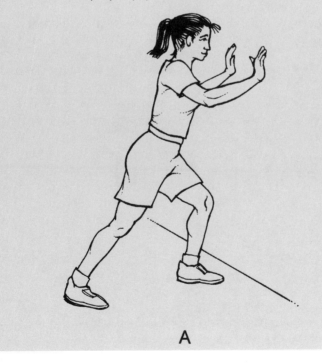

A

FIGURE 7-3 Heel cord stretching exercises.

B. As illustrated, stand on the edge of a stair. While supporting your-self well with your hands on the banister, keep your knees straight and drop your heels, stretching your heel cords.

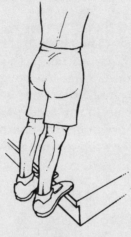

B

C. As illustrated, holding onto the top of a table, lean forward with your knees bent and your heels flat on the floor. You should feel your heel cords stretching.

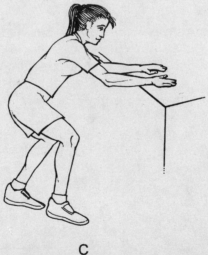

C

All of these exercises should be performed with 6 repetitions, hold-ing each position of stretch for a slow count of 6.

FIGURE 7-3   (continued)

Treatment of tendo-achillis and retrocalcaneal (behind the heel bone) bursitis is with ice, rest, and an oral antiinflammatory drug. An appropriate pad to unload the heel during weight bearing is prescribed, and local injections of steroid are given sometimes.

TOE PROBLEMS

Hammertoes are produced by a muscle imbalance that causes the end joints of one of the smaller toes to bend down while the closer joint bends up. The joints tend to stiffen permanently in this position. Hammertoes can be inherited or may be caused by a nervous system abnormality. The condition is aggravated by tight-fitting shoes that result in an uncomfortable callus at the tip of the toe and a painful corn where it is angulated upward and presses on the toe box of the shoe. The deformity is called a hammertoe because it looks like one of the hammers that strike the strings in a piano. It is distinguished from a "mallet toe," in which the bent toe joint is the one near the tip.

Proper treatment is surgical, consisting of either removal of bone and lengthening of tendons or fusing the involved toe joint(s). This usually can be performed on an outpatient basis under local anesthesia. Recovery is within three to six weeks. In cases in which surgery is contraindicated for whatever reason, the patient can use an open shoe or have footwear custom-made to conform to the shape of the foot. Such a shoe is called a "space boot," and although it is not particularly attractive, it is very comfortable. Whereas the standard shoe expects the foot to conform to its shape, the space boot is designed to fit only one pair of feet. A cast of the foot is taken, and a custom shoe is fashioned on a last made from the cast. "Space boots" usually are oxfords. They are fabricated from very supple leather (often deerskin) and have cushioned soles and a supporting insert made of light plastic foam. They close on the side by laces or Velcro and are very light and comfortable to wear.

BUNIONS

The scientific name for a bunion is *hallux valgus* (great toe—bent in). This deformity is more common in women than in men and tends to run in families. Bunions are *de rigeur* for ballet dancers, an adaptation to the constricting *en point* slippers into which they force their feet. Some principal ballet dancers, such as Suzanne Farrell of the New York City Ballet, can use 350 pairs of toe shoes in a season. An unsightly bump develops at the base of the big toe, where the joint angles inward. The width of the forefoot is increased and the bunion is irritated where it pushes against the shoe. An inflamed bursa can form beneath the skin at this point. As the bunion deformity progresses, it forces the second toe into an overlapping hammertoe position. People who have rheumatoid arthritis or flat feet are more prone to develop bunions. Cramming the foot into a narrow pointed toe box with a high heel will aggravate the condition.

Wide shoes and soft toe supports (bunion posts) as well as warm foot soaks, over-the-counter analgesics, and whirlpool baths are some conservative ways of treating bunions. The definitive care is surgical. An operation called a bunionectomy is performed in a hospital setting. This may entail a spinal or general anesthetic. Surgery involves removing the bunion bump and realigning the great toe. This often requires correcting the deformity by cutting the bone and resetting it in the straightened position. Soft tissue reconstruction of ligaments that have been stretched out of shape also may be necessary.

Resecting the bone of the bunion joint is another surgical alternative that removes the focus of arthritic irritation. Yet another option is to replace the involved joint with a prosthetic implant that acts as a joint filler, usually fabricated from the bio-inert polymer Silastic or other plastic or from the metal titanium. This keeps the bone separated and properly aligned, maintaining the length of the toe but still allowing toe flexibility.

Rehabilitation after bunion surgery can be prolonged. Although the patient often can walk immediately in a plaster cast in a special shoe after cast removal, it may take as long as three months for healing to be complete and for standing and walking in a normal fashion to become possible.

A *bunionette* (or tailor's bunion), so called because tailors used to sit cross-legged on the floor, which irritated the outer margins of their feet, is an outer angulation at the base of the fifth toe that produces a painful bump. Surgical removal of the bony prominence is a simple procedure that can be performed on an outpatient basis, does not require a cast, and is safe and usually effective.

Hallux rigidus is rigidity of the great toe characterized by swelling, pain, and sometimes redness at the base of the toe, but there is no angulation or bump as in a bunion. This condition is due to arthritis at the base of the toe, which may result from either a single injury or repeated stress. It sometimes responds to oral antiinflammatory medication and a steroid injection. Wearing a shoe that has a rigid sole or using a special splint may prevent excess motion at this joint, decreasing pain. Surgery involves removal of one surface of the joint. Resurfacing with a prosthetic implant is sometimes performed.

TRANSVERSE ARCH COLLAPSE

Pressure on the transverse arch can cause its collapse, with painful callosities forming under the second, third, and fourth metatarsal heads (metatarsalgia). A metatarsal pad placed in the shoe just behind the metatarsal heads or a metatarsal bar fixed to the sole of the shoe can help reduce further pressure. Wearing high-heeled shoes should be avoided. Sometimes it is necessary to surgically provide a sling support of tissue (i.e., fascia) for the arch.

CLUBFOOT

Clubfoot is a common congenital deformity (about 1–2 per 1,000 live births) that occurs more frequently in boys and is bilateral (both sides) in 33 percent of cases. The medical term is *congenital talipes equinovarus*. The term *talipes* means clubfoot. The foot is pointed down and out, like a horse's foot (hence "equino"). The forefoot is shifted medially and twisted in (varus). Broadly speaking, and with some overlap, there are two types of clubfoot: (1) *intrinsic clubfoot*, which is due to an inborn structural defect of the foot, and (2) *extrinsic clubfoot*, in which the deformity occurs because of malposition during fetal growth. You might guess that the intrinsic type is more difficult to treat and most frequently requires surgery for correction.

Clubfoot usually is detected at birth, and treatment with serial manipulations and casts to bring the foot and ankle into the corrected position can be started immediately. It is necessary to change casts on a weekly basis to accommodate growth. If full correction has not been achieved at six weeks, operative correction is necessary. This consists of release of soft tissue and tendons, making it possible to bring the foot into a normal attitude. Surgery is followed by casting for approximately six weeks. After casts are removed, special shoes are worn to prevent the deformity from recurring. Such support usually continues for at least several years. An experimental treatment involves the injection of botulinum toxin (the highly refined neurotoxin from the bacteria *Clostridium botulinum*, which causes food poisoning and muscle paralysis) into contracted foot muscles. When combined with vigorous physical therapy (stretching), these injections have expedited correction of clubfoot deformity.

RHEUMATOID ARTHRITIS

Rheumatoid arthritis, which can inflame joints throughout the body, often starts in the feet and ankles. Conservative treatment consists of appropriate medication, a program of foot care, and custom-made shoes. Reconstructive surgery, such as removal of deformed metatarsal joints, is available for the severely involved foot.

OSTEOARTHRITIS

Degenerative arthritis can affect any joint(s) in the foot but most commonly involves the joint of the big toe, causing hallux rigidus. Surgical treatment includes partial resection or reconstructing the joint.

GOUT

Gout usually attacks the big toe (podagra) and is caused by too much uric acid in the body. This condition is covered in detail in Chapter 2 (see pages 24–26).

CONCLUSION

The German poet Goethe said that "a pretty foot's a great gift of nature." Be that as it may, a comfortable foot is a "joy forever." We tend to take our feet for granted until they begin to hurt and remind us how important they are to our well-being. Your feet will remain your friends if you develop an awareness of the value of foot care and follow some simple procedures, such as wearing properly fitted shoes and hose, employing daily foot hygiene, and seeking professional help when self-care of a foot problem proves inadequate.

SIX RULES TO KEEP YOU ON YOUR FEET

1. Bathe your feet at least once a day for ten minutes in warm water and follow with a brisk cold cream massage.

2. Use alternating foot baths of warm and cold water, starting and ending in the warm water, spending two minutes in the warm and then one minute in the cold for a period of eleven minutes.

3. Rest your feet whenever you can. When sitting, cross your legs and rest your feet on their outside borders. When possible, lie down and elevate you feet higher than the rest of your body.

4. Exercise your feet frequently by wiggling the toes vigorously, moving your ankle and foot up and down, in and out. Try to pick up a pencil, clothespin, or marbles with the toes, or attempt to crumple a small piece of light paper or a washrag.

5. Wear proper foot wear. Be sure your shoes are well fitted and wide and long enough for comfort.

6. Pare your toenails properly, in a straight line and relatively long. Sand any calluses with a pumice stone during the bath or a fine emery board when dry.

CASE REPORT—THE FOOT

Al and Jane were not concerned when they noticed that their son Jeff had flatfeet. After all, he was an otherwise normal child who started to walk just after his first birthday. Al and Jane realized that many infants have flatfeet, which is due to a thick fat pad and general joint laxity. However, Jeff's feet remained flat as he grew and lost his baby fat. He was examined by his pediatrician. Tight heel cords are a common cause of flatfeet in childhood and Jeff's heel cords were a little tight, but he did not complain of pain. It was decided to observe the condition further. In early adolescence Jeff's feet began to hurt. He had difficulty participating in running sports and would take his shoes off as soon as he got home, complaining of pain in his feet. Jeff was referred to an orthopaedic surgeon, who examined his feet and found limited motion in the joint between the talus and calcaneus. A special X-ray revealed an abnormal fusion between these joints, which was further identified by a CT scan. The lack of motion at this joint was imposing increased stress on adjacent joints, causing pain and peroneal muscle spasm. Untreated, this ultimately might cause degenerative arthritis. Such fusions may occur in one or both feet and equally in both sexes. They often are familial and, on close inquiry, Jeff's parents found that there was a family history of painful feet in several cousins.

Jeff's feet were treated with short walking casts for a month. When the casts were removed, the feet were free of discomfort for a short while, but the pain eventually came back. An operation was performed in which the coalition (fusion) was resected (removed) and fat and muscle were interposed between the bones to prevent recurrence. This was successful in Jeff's case, and although he never became an Olympic track star or a professional basketball player, he was able to conduct his normal daily activities, including recreational activities, without discomfort.

QUESTIONS AND ANSWERS—THE FOOT

Q: Why are the soles of the feet so ticklish?

A: The soles of the feet, like the armpits, have a large concentration of nerve endings, which makes these areas very sensitive. That's why they are so ticklish.

Q: What are the best shoes for "seniors?"

A: A shoe, such as a topsider or boating shoe, with a relatively thin, hard rubber sole is best for maintaining balance. Athletic shoes with spongy soles are the worst kind because it is more difficult to judge the angle of your foot in relation to the ground with a thick, cushiony shoe. This can lead to loss of balance and falling.

Q: Why do women have a different gait than men?

A: Women have a wider pelvis, a different angle of their hips, more knock-knee, and increased flatness of their hind feet. These factors help keep the plumb line of the body centered. Additionally, women have narrower heels and shorter legs relative to their height. Competitive female runners are predominantly midfoot strikers as compared with male "heel strikers." They also strike the ground more often for the same distance, generating more ground reaction forces.

Q: When is it safe to let a child taking ballet lessons go "on point?"

A: Many ballet teachers allow a child to toe-dance based on his or her individual talent. Others refuse to put a student "on point" until a certain age, most frequently given as 12 years. However, this depends on having significant training, and it may be that with such instruction a child considerably younger is ready to go on his or her toes. Some children should never go on their toes, whereas others seem to be born with the ability to perform "on point." In the final analysis, trust in the ballet instructor's judgment probably is the most important variable in deciding when a student should go "on point."

Q: Do some feet have extra bones?

A: A number of common accessory ossification centers (small extra bones) are found in otherwise normal feet. These are seldom symptomatic except for an accessory tarsal navicular bone, which can be painful.

Q: What is polydactyly? Syndactyly?

A: Polydactyly (many—fingers) is a developmental anomaly characterized by the presence of supernumerary digits (fingers or toes). It is the most common congenital anomaly of the hand or foot. Syndactyly (together—fingers) is marked by the persistence of webbing between adjacent fingers or toes. These conditions are more common in females and in Blacks and sometimes are inherited as an autosomal dominant trait. Corrective surgery is available.

Q: Why do some children walk on their toes?

A: Toe-walking may occur in otherwise normal children, but it is common in children with neuromuscular disorders because of weakness and contracture (tightening) of the heel cord.

Q: Why are very high heels bad for the feet?

A: When standing or walking barefooted or in flat shoes, you normally bear 60 percent of your weight on your heels and 40 percent on your forefoot and toes. Wearing a modest (e.g., "little Louis") heel in an otherwise well-balanced shoe is of little consequence. Wearing high, spiked heels loads your heels with only 20 to 40 percent of your weight, causing your forefoot to bear the remaining 60 to 80 percent. When the toes are jammed with that much force into a narrow toe box, the stage is set for the development of hammertoes, metatarsalgia, bunions, and the like.

We've now completed our journey through the joints of your legs. Let's now examine the joints of your arms. But on the way we have to take a look at your neck and then your spine.

8

The Neck

You should show first the spine of the neck
with its tendons like the mast of a ship...
Leonardo daVinci
Quaderni D'Anatomia
Vol II

One of the first places in which pain occurs as a result of stress is the neck. It is no mere coincidence that people often somaticize tension to the neck. Our organ language reflects this in the common complaint "he or she is a pain in the neck." Because the neck is the gateway, as it were, to the shoulders and arms in one direction and the head in the other direction, difficulties that originate in the neck can result in symptoms such as headache (usually in the rear or occipital area), dizziness or nausea, pain or cramping in the arms, and tingling or numbness in the fingers.

Like the vertebrae of the back, those of the neck are separated by pads of fibrocartilage, called discs, which act as shock absorbers. Also like the vertebrae of the back, those of the neck contain joints (facets) that permit significant motion, including 180° of rotation, approximately 120° of tilt to either side, and almost 90° of forward (flexion) and backward (extension) bending. One of the strongest hinge joints in the body connects the base of the skull with the first cervical (neck) vertebra. Most mammals have the same seven neck bones we do, even the giraffe, whose neck can reach over six feet in length.

"Thy neck is as a tower of ivory..." sighs the lover in the Song of Songs (Solomon VII, 4), and indeed elongation of the neck is considered a sign of female beauty and status by some African tribes. This is accomplished by stacking metal rings on

129

a girl's neck during growth. In this way, the neck is not lengthened so much as the girls shoulders are depressed, giving the appearance of elongation, sometimes by 50 percent or more.

ANATOMY

Anatomists called the topmost vertebra the *atlas* after the Titan in Greek mythology who was condemned to carry the earth and heavens on his shoulders. The atlas, supporting the skull, does not have the solid body of bone that is typical of the other vertebrae. Rather, it forms a bony ring with a large central opening. Rounded projections off the skull's occipital bone (the bone making up much of the skull's base) fit into two large hollows on top of the atlas. Tough ligaments bind the cranium to the atlas. Beneath the atlas another vertebra called the *axis* sends a bony projection through the opening in the atlas. This articulation permits the atlas, holding the skull, to rotate.

Your head is supported by the seven cervical vertebrae and is held in place by 32 complex muscles. Eight nerves exiting from the spinal cord conduct impulses for movement and sensation (including pain) to and from the head, upper body, and arms. Four major arteries and veins carry blood between the head and the heart as they course through the neck.

The delicate spinal cord runs through the center of the stacked cervical vertebrae and is protected by them. The cervical nerves, like branches of a tree, exit through small holes in the side of the vertebrae called *foramina* (Figure 8-1).

MOVEMENT

The neck has to move more than any other part of the spine, which makes it more vulnerable to injury and degenerative diseases. Its muscles and ligaments continuously hold the head up and also allow it to move in three basic ways, with countless combinations. You can bend your head forward or backward on your neck. You can rotate your head to either side. You also can tilt your head to either side. If something goes wrong in the neck, the effects can be far-reaching. Pain originating in the neck may be felt in other areas, such as the scalp, ears, face,

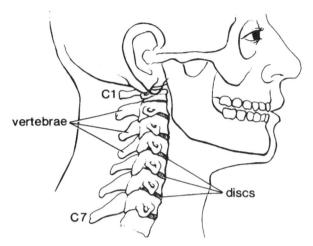

FIGURE 8-1 The cervical spine.

arms, shoulders, hands, fingers, or occasionally even in the chest. This is called *referred pain*.

NECK PAIN

In addition to tension, neck pain can occur from chronic malposture. Your head weighs 15 pounds, and you can imagine what happens to body awareness if the neck muscles are held contracted to support a poorly balanced head. Other causes of neck pain include arthritis (either osteoarthritis or inflammatory arthritis), any disease process involving bone (tumor, infection, and the like), or accidents that cause strains and sprains. Fractures or dislocations are more serious injuries. These can occur during athletic contact, industrial mishaps, or automobile collisions.

CHILDREN

Neck pain is uncommon in children and almost always has an organic basis. Acute *torticollis* can force the head to tilt to one side because of muscle spasm. This can be caused by inflammation of the lymph nodes of the neck or by minor displacement of a cervical vertebra. It usually resolves spontaneously, and treatment is symptomatic, including rest while immobilizing the neck with a folded towel.

Infantile muscular torticollis is due to an organizing hematoma (collection of blood) in one of the neck muscles (usually the sternocleidomastoid). This causes the muscle to shorten and contract, and the head tilts to one side. The tight muscle can often be stretched with a brace or a cast, but sometimes excision of the mass is necessary for cure.

Congenital abnormalities of the neck include a variety of conditions in which there are anomalies or fusions of the cervical vertebrae or associated bones.

Instability of the axis is rare and usually is due to a congenital bony defect or marked ligamentous laxity as seen in Down's syndrome (mongolism).

ADULTS

Whiplash

The common "whiplash" injury (in which the neck is "cracked" like a whip) usually happens when a standing automobile is struck from behind or an accelerating vehicle hits a solid object. In either case, because of the sudden impact, the head keeps moving and, as it passes rapidly over the stationary neck, in either hyperextension (backward) or hyperflexion (forward) motion, the vertebrae are compressed. This can cause the neck to accept a compression force of well over 500 pounds, which may result in ligamentous or bony damage. Discomfort includes pain, often referred to the shoulder or arm, as well as nausea, dizziness (which may be secondary to injury of the blood vessels), headache, and persistent neck stiffness.

Most whiplash injuries, like other sprains, respond to conservative treatment, including moist heat, the use of an appropriate soft or semirigid myocervical collar support, cervical traction (either intermittent or continuous), special cervical pillows, diathermy (deep electrical heat) and massage, a transepidermal nerve stimulation (TENS) unit, and appropriate antipain medication (anodynes) or nonsteroidal antiinflammatory drugs (NSAIDs).

Because the spine is like the axle of a vehicle, it cannot be malaligned at one end without causing trouble at the other end. Proper posture is very important to ensure not only a healthy back but also a healthy and pain-free neck. Any job or hobby that requires a lot of leaning tends to stress the neck. Frequent relief of this strain by changing position and using neck stretching and strengthening exercises will go a long way toward preventing common neck problems secondary to postural malalignment or emotional tension.

ISOMETRIC EXERCISES FOR THE NECK

These exercises can strengthen the neck. They are particularly useful for someone weaning himself from a neck collar.

The head moves in six directions on the neck: (1) forward, (2) backward, (3) tilting to the right, (4) tilting to the left, (5) rotating to the right, and (6) rotating to the left.

Restraining motion of the head by linking the hands and placing them on the forehead, attempt to move the head by forcing it against the hands to a slow count of six. Relax.

Now place the linked hands behind the head and repeat the exercise attempting to force the head backwards. Remember to use maximum strength to a slow count of six. Relax.

Use the right hand to restrain the head from tilting to the right as you repeat the exercise as above.

Now use the left hand, blocking a forceful attempt to tilt the head to the left. Remember to use maximum strength to a slow count of six. Relax.

Finally, restrain rotation to the right by cupping the right hand under the chin. Forcefully attempt to rotate the head to the right again to a slow count of six. Relax.

Repeat the attempt to rotate the head, this time to the left while using the left hand cupped under the left side of the chin as a restraint.

Remember, these are isometric exercises that rely on a forceful muscle contraction. You must exert at least 75 percent of maximal muscle force for any benefit. The head and neck must be kept in line and upright facing forward and should not move during the exercise. This training regimen is designed to strengthen all the muscles of the neck. The entire exercise program takes less than one minute. It should be performed three times a day.

Arthritis

Wear and tear processes (spondylosis), such as those found in arthritic joints, can affect the bones and joints of the neck. This typically is seen in areas in which most motion in the neck occurs, usually at the level of the fourth through sixth cervical vertebrae. Arthritis or disc disease in the neck may require treatment similar to that for these conditions elsewhere in the spine (see Chapter 9). This includes the occasional necessity for an operation such as fusion of several vertebrae or decompression by removing bone and/or a protruding or herniated disc that is pinching a nerve.

Muscle spasm can be relieved by the application of moist heat; deep massage; relaxing medications; cold, which can ease a small muscle spasm or "knot"; or injections of local anesthetic into triggerpoints.

Any neck problem that does not readily respond to simple conservative home treatment should be referred to your doctor, who will take a history and perform a physical examination. This will include a thorough neurologic study of the head and neck, shoulders, and arms. X-rays and occasionally a blood test may be ordered. Special tests, including CT and MRI, electrical examinations (EMG—electromyogram of the muscles; and NCV—assessment of nerve conduction velocity) can help decide whether pressure on the nerves is the cause of pain.

The "wall test" is a way of checking your neck posture. Stand with your back to a smooth wall. Keep your heels several inches from the wall. Your buttocks and shoulders should touch the wall. The back of your head should be close to the wall. Keeping your chin level, walk away and then return to check your position. Try, in a relaxed way, to carry your head and neck in this posture all day long.

Pain

Geographically, there are two types of pain. There is *local pain*, which is experienced by the patient at the site of pain causation, for instance, pain from bruising caused by a blow on the arm. *Referred pain* is pain perceived to be in a location a distance from the structure at fault. Referred pain can be divided into the following categories:

1. *nerve root pain*, a shooting-type pain with clearly defined borders, usually accompanied by a "pins and needles" sensation;
2. *somatic referred pain*, which is referred from structures within the musculoskeletal system other than the nerve root; somatic referred pain is a deep, boring ache that is diffuse in distribution; and
3. *visceral referred pain*, which arises from a disorder of an internal organ such as the heart that refers pain down the left arm, or the gallbladder, which refers pain to the back; this tends to be diffuse in nature and can be confused with somatic referred pain. Nerve root and somatic referred pain are increased or decreased with movement, but visceral pain remains unchanged. Any of the soft tissue or bony structures of the neck (or the rest of the spine), including the discs, all ligaments, all muscles, all joint capsules, and all bony structures, as well as blood vessels, can give rise to pain.

Cervical Disc Lesions

Treatment of a problem with a cervical disc is similar to that of a lumbar disc (see next chapter, The Spine).

Acute Torticollis

This is a twisted or wry neck and is treated with hot packs, rest, neck support, and medications to relieve pain and muscle spasm.

Cervical Joint Lock

Cervical joint lock shares certain similarities with acute torticollis but is more serious because it is due to a sudden movement of the cervical spine that traps a meniscoid structure (pad of fibrocartilage) between the articular surfaces of one of the cervical facet joints. It can be diagnosed by X-ray and treated with longitudinal traction and/or careful manipulation to unlock the cervical spine.

After determining the specific reason for your pain, your doctor will prescribe a neck care program tailored to your needs. This can include frequent periods of rest with a special supportive neck

NECK STRETCHING EXERCISES

1. Sit well back in straight back chair, feet hooked inside around front chair legs.

2. Rotate head, neck, and body to the right as far as possible.

3. Bring left arm across chest and grasp chair along right side of body.

4. Place palm of right hand around left side of tip of closed jaw.

5. Now pull with left arm and push jaw with right hand at the same time as much as can be tolerated.

6. Do this for ten seconds and then relax. Repeat five times.

7. Now rotate to the left, reverse arms, and stretch neck to the left as above.

pillow. A soft or firm cervical collar may be advised. Home traction is another simple method of relieving pressure by taking the strain off the neck muscles. This typically is applied with the neck in slight flexion and the chin tilted forward as this is the proper neck posture for the patient with neck pain. Acute muscle spasm can be relieved by ice. Chronic pain or spasm often will respond to moist heat (bath, shower, hot water bottle, hot compress, or moist heating pad). The vicious cycle of pain and muscle spasm that occurs with chronic neck problems often can be interrupted by an injection of local anesthetic or cortisone into triggerpoints of pain. Massage can help, as can exercises that stretch the neck muscles.

A more formal way of applying these treatments is through physical therapy. The therapist may apply heat using deep electrical diathermy or moist heat packs. Intermittent traction can be administered with a motorized unit. The patient usually is instructed in appropriate range of motion exercises to increase neck mobility. Isometric workouts will strengthen the neck muscles. An occupational therapist can review the patient's lifestyle and methods for handling tasks of daily living and recommend ways and means to avoid neck strain at home and on the job.

Just remember that you do not have to put up with neck tension and pain. By following a simple program that includes proper posture, relaxation, increasing range of motion, and strengthening of your neck, you can develop a strong, well-balanced neck and avoid the recurrent pain and stiffness that accompanies the neglected neck syndrome.

CASE REPORT—The Neck

Mary L. was a 36-year-old secretary. After a minor traffic accident she experienced right-sided neck pain that went into her right shoulder and down her right arm to her elbow. She also complained of tingling in the fourth and fifth fingers of her right hand and difficulty finding a comfortable position in which to sleep. Mary tried several over-the-counter pain medications and applied heat to her neck and shoulder. This did not provide lasting relief, so she consulted her doctor.

Examination revealed that Mary had limited motion in her neck with pain on rotation and extension (backward motion) of her head on her neck. She had diminished sensation to touch and pinprick in her hand, her biceps deep tendon reflex was depressed at the elbow, and her grip strength was reduced. An X-ray revealed narrowing of the space between her fourth and fifth and fifth and sixth cervical vertebrae, indicating pathology of the intervertebral discs at these levels. A subsequent MRI examination confirmed protrusion of the discs to the right, pressing on the nerves to the arm. An electromyogram was abnormal, and a diagnosis of cervical disc protrusion with radiculitis (inflammation of the root of a spinal nerve) was made.

Treatment of Mary's condition included an NSAID and the use of a soft cervical collar to relieve the neck muscles supporting her head. Physical therapy, including ultrasound, heat, massage, and cervical traction, was prescribed. Mary was instructed in how to avoid further strain to her neck and purchased a pillow that supported her neck to use at night. Subsequently she was given reconditioning exercises for her neck, and continues to improve on this regimen. It is doubtful that she will require surgical excision of the offending intervertebral discs with a local fusion of the unstable vertebrae; however, only time will tell.

QUESTIONS AND ANSWERS—THE NECK

Q: What is "wry neck?"

A: Wry neck is torticollis, literally, a twisted neck (torque, to twist; collum, neck—both from the Latin). This may occur spontaneously following minimal trauma or after a respiratory infection. Tilting of the head probably is due to muscle spasm secondary to cervical lymphadenitis (inflammation of the lymph glands of the neck) or a minor displacement of the cervical vertebrae. Acute torticollis usually resolves spontaneously in one to two days. The deformity often disappears as abruptly as it began. The neck can be immobilized with a folded towel and heat can be applied.

Other common causes of stiff neck are from sleeping in an awkward position, exposing the neck to an unusual temperature change (such as direct air conditioning), or sustaining a sudden twist or jar. If it persists beyond a week in a child, acute torticollis is called "rotatory displacement." This condition requires treatment to prevent permanent fixation and residual deformity related to subluxation (slipping) of a cervical vertebra. Imaging with X-ray and CT may document the displacement, and traction can reduce it. Repositioning and fusion of the vertebrae may be required for displacements that persist longer than a month. Severe spastic torticollis can be treated with injections of Botox®, a dilute solution of botulinum toxin that paralyzes the nerve relaxing the muscles of the neck.

Q: How can I protect my neck during daily activity?
A: 1. Do not tilt your head back when washing or shaving.

2. Wash your hair in the shower instead of in the sink.
3. Use a headrest to support your head while driving.
4. Avoid prolonged driving and make regular stops to rest.
5. Take frequent breaks during work and leisure activities.
6. Try not to sleep on your stomach. It is better for your neck to sleep on your side or back.

Q: Are "slipped discs" as common in the neck as they are in the low back?
A: The anatomy of the cervical vertebrae is such that the edge of the bone curves slightly, producing a restraining barrier to protrusion of the disc. Also, the neck is not commonly subjected to the magnitude of forces that load the lumbar spine. Therefore, slipped discs are not as common in the neck as they are in the lower back.

Like the popular song says, "The neck bone is connected to the spine bone... ," so we'll now proceed to look at the rest of the spinal column.

9

The Spine

The spine is a series of bones running down your back.
You sit on one end of it and your head sits on the other.

Anonymous

Ever since humans assumed an erect posture there has been a
need for adaptation and development from the skeletal arrangement seen in quadripeds (four-legged animals). The very form of
the human spine is due to some of these adaptations and
changes. Knowing how a healthy spine works may help you
understand how moving wisely can protect your back and keep
it free of pain.

CONFIGURATION

The *vertebral column* is a spiral spring in the form of the letter
"S." A newborn child has a relatively straight backbone. Curves
develop to support functions that include holding up the trunk,
serving as an anchor for the extremities, and keeping the head
erect. The S-curvature enables the vertebral column to absorb
the shocks of walking. A straight spine would conduct the jarring shocks directly from the pelvic girdle to the head. In the
quadriped, the viscera hang from the spine. In erect animals
such as humans, who have a straight spinal column, the spine
would be pulled forward by the viscera. Curvature solves this
problem by providing additional space for the viscera to sit within the concavities of the thoracic and pelvic regions.

The distribution of weight throughout the entire body is affected by the spine's S-curvature. To a large extent, the upper sector carries the head, the central sector the thoracic viscera (the organs and structures in the chest), and the lower sector the abdominal viscera. If the column were straight, this weight load would increase from the head downward and be relatively great at the base. Finally, the bent spring arrangement of the S-curvature renders the spine far less vulnerable to breakage than a straight column would.

ANATOMY

The spine is built of 33 small bones, the *vertebrae*, bodily segmentation having already occurred in earlier "nonvertebrate" life forms such as the earthworm. The seven cervical vertebrae in the neck are the smallest and allow the greatest range of movement. The thoracic vertebrae, 12 heavier bones, lie beneath them, forming the upper back. The thoracic vertebrae also hold the ribs in place. Special disc-shaped indentations called the *rib facets* help anchor the ribs on both sides of the vertebrae. Five lumbar vertebrae make up the small of the back and are the largest bones of the spine, as they bear most of the body's weight. Beneath these, five smaller bones, which are separate at birth, fuse at about age 25 to form the wedge-shaped sacrum ("sacred bone"), which fits between the hips. The last segment of the spine is a small tapering bone built of four fused rudimentary vertebrae, the residuum of a tail and without any function, called the coccyx (Gr. cuckoo—whose bill it is said to resemble) (Figure 9-1). The coccyx sometimes is fractured or irritated and may even require excision.

All the vertebrae are similar structurally, with the exception of the fused vertebrae in the sacrum and coccyx and the first and second cervical vertebrae. The main portion of a vertebra is called the *body*. It is a flattened oval block of bone. Short columns called the *pedicles* arise from the back of the body. Small plates called *lamina* seal the opening between the two pedicles, creating a circular channel through which the spinal cord passes. Three winglike extensions emanate from the lamina. Spaced at a 90-degree angle from each other, they anchor muscles and give the spine its knobby appearance under the skin. The *articular*

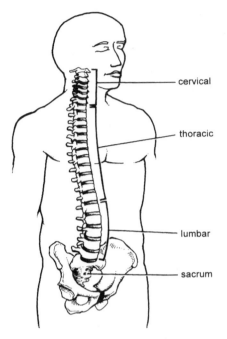

cervical

thoracic

lumbar

sacrum

FIGURE 9-1   Anatomy of your spine.

processes, two smooth nubs on top of the vertebrae and two beneath, are called the *vertebral facets*. These link each vertebra with its neighbors above and below (Figure 9-2).

MOVEMENT

A high degree of protection for the central nervous system is made possible by the relatively small amount of movement permitted by the component parts of the vertebral column. The spinal cord is enclosed in the back and on the sides and is protected by the part of each vertebra called the neural arch. Between the neural arches are sheaths of elastic connective tissue, the *ligamenta flava* (white ligaments). Here, some protective function is sacrificed for the sake of motion because forward bending of part of the spinal column leads to separation between the lamina and between the spines of the neural arches of adjoining vertebrae. It is through the ligamenta flava of the lower lumbar region (the small of the back) that the needle in

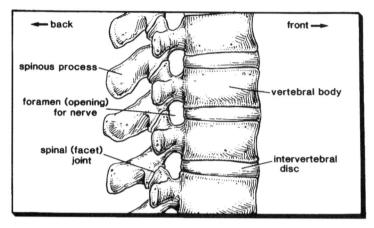

FIGURE 9-2   Normal vertebrae.

the procedure of lumbar puncture enters the subarachnoid space, in which spinal fluid circulates around the spinal cord.

The vertebral column is also important in the anchoring of muscles. Many of the muscles attached to it move various segments of the back. Some are superficial, whereas others are deep. The anchoring function of the spinal column is important for muscles that arise on the trunk, in whole or in part from the column or from ligaments attached to it, and then are inserted onto the bones of the arms and legs.

VERTEBRAL DISCS

Between each vertebra there is special padding that in total occupies about one-fourth of an adult spine. The padding is in the form of *discs* that act as buffers against the shocks applied to the spine by stress such as running and jumping, and prevent the bones from grinding against each other. They also permit motion between the vertebrae, bolstering the spine with added strength as well as flexibility. These discs play a role in shaping the spinal column as it rests at the body's vertical center of gravity. As we have seen, the spine crosses the gravity line, weaving back and forth. To create spinal curvature, the discs subtly change shape, with portions narrowing or widening so that the vertebrae do not sit directly on top of each other.

There are 23 *intervertebral discs*, one between each vertebral pair below the first cervical and two above the second sacral
vertebra. The lower back (lumbar) discs are thickest, the chest
(thoracic) discs are thinnest, and the neck (cervical) discs are of
intermediate size. These differences reflect the function of the
discs in each area.

FACETS

If the intervertebral discs were the only joints between the vertebrae, the backbone could move in any direction. However, each
pair of vertebrae with an intervertebral disc also has a pair of
synovial joints, called vertebral facet joints, one of which lies on
each side of the vertebral neural arch. Depending on their angulation, these joints limit the kinds of independent movement
possible between the vertebrae. The thoracic vertebrae move in
only two directions, the lumbar vertebrae move in only three
directions, whereas the cervical vertebrae below the atlas have
full freedom of movement.

STANDING

The distinctive shape of the spine is evidence of its adaptation
to the human's erect stance. There are many advantages to
bipedalism (two-footed walking). Most significant is freeing the
hands for tasks more complicated than bearing weight, which
led to an increase in the size of the human brain. The history of
the spine's adaptation to bipedalism is reflected in the experience of every child learning to hold his head upright, to pull
himself forward, to crawl, and, finally, to walk. The spinal column responds to new demands at each stage in this sequence.

The spine of the infant is C-shaped, with its vertebrae still
largely undifferentiated. The cervical curve starts to form when
the infant attempts to hold up his or her head. The cervical
curve is fully formed by about four months of age, when this
task has been mastered. It is, however, the least marked of the
spinal curves. The most pronounced curve, and the one unique
to humans, is the lumbar curve, a concave bend in the lower
back that begins to develop when the child first tries to walk. By

the age of two his or her first unbalanced steps gradually yield to a confident stride as the lumbar curve deepens and balance improves.

The spinal column is an expressive instrument. If your body is stiff and rigid, or collapsed and limp, your mind will follow suit. Our language is full of phrases that demonstrate this relationship. Like a cat arching its back in fear, human posture reflects feelings. Depression, submission, happiness, and authority all can be easily read in the slope and posture of the back. We say, "He won't change his position on this issue" or "The company has taken an aggressive stance on that question." The bible refers to the Hebrews as a "stiff-necked people."

Shakespeare's King Richard III had a grossly misshapen back. A malevolant presence in two of Shakespeare's plays, Richard's character is more twisted than his body. Shakespeare made Richard's spinal deformity the source of his discontent as well as a symbol of his evil. Richard mourned, "Why, love foreswore me in my mother's womb ... to make an envious mountain on my back ... where sits deformity to mock my body...."

SPINAL CURVES

Although essential for the health of the back and the body, spinal curves are crippling when exaggerated. Extreme lateral (to the side) curvature, called *scoliosis*, warps posture and upsets the body's balance. *Lordosis* (swayback) is an abnormal concave curvature of the spine, usually in the lumbar region. *Kyphosis* (hunchback) is an accentuated convex curvature of the thoracic vertebrae.

The ribs connect directly to the thoracic vertebrae. Twelve pairs of ribs spring from the sides of these vertebrae, their heads nestled into shallow facets. The upper seven pairs are true ribs that arch around the body and attach to the sternum (breastbone) via shafts of cartilage (costal cartilage). The remaining five pairs of ribs are "false" because they link with the sternum indirectly. The lower two pairs of false ribs "float," barely hovering about the side of the body. They do not connect at all with the sternum but instead terminate in cartilage connected to muscle of the abdominal wall.

As mentioned before, the intervertebral discs are the cushions in your spine. Each has a spongy center (nucleus pulposus) and a tougher outer ring (annulus) that contains pain fibers. The nucleus is a transparent jelly containing 88 percent water. Fluid movement within the nucleus allows the vertebrae to rock back and forth on the discs, giving you the flexibility to bend and move. Your discs fill with fluid and press against the annulus while you sleep. In the morning, upon awakening, the annulus is taut and less flexible. This is why sudden movements in the morning can cause injuries to your disc. During the day fluid is pushed in and out of the nucleus, nourishing your discs as you move. Loss of fluid makes you shorter at the end of the day by approximately one inch. In the evening your annulus is more flexible, making injury less likely. With aging, the disc loses some of its capacity to absorb water, which explains the permanent loss of flexibility and height in later years.

THE CHILD'S SPINE

According to a recent review, low back pain can affect up to 30 percent of children, with the greatest incidence after age 13. If pain occurs at night or lasts several weeks in children younger than 11 years and is accompanied by stiffness in the legs, fever, loss of sensation or weakness, or if it interferes with play, sports, or school attendance, a serious problem is likely.

There are many possible causes of back pain in children: inflammatory, infectious, traumatic, tumor, neurologic, developmental, congenital, and psychogenic. Even the use of a heavy backpack can be a cause of pain. Any child complaining of back pain should be taken seriously, and an appropriate examination should be conducted.

The child's spine usually is evaluated as a part of a screening examination or to assess pain or deformity. Imaging studies (X-ray, CT, bone scan, MRI) may be indicated to make a definitive diagnosis.

Back pain may be due to (1) *discitis* (disc infection characterized by fever, limp, and severe pain, and treated by rest and intravenous antibiotics, although surgical drainage of the infected area sometimes is necessary); (2) *stress fracture*. In the low lumbar spine this may present as *spondylolisthesis*, a fracture or elongation of the pars interarticularis (that part of the vertebral lamina [arch] that connects the superior [upper] and inferior [lower] articular facets), allowing forward slipping of the vertebra. Simple disjunction of the pars without slippage is called *spondylolysis*. It presents with back pain and limited range of motion. Oblique X-rays of the lumbosacral spine reveal the defect. Treatment is by bracing and/or surgery (fusion of the offending vertebrae).

Both benign and malignant tumors can involve the spinal column. A common benign tumor is the *osteoid osteoma*. Patients typically complain of night pain relieved by aspirin. Treatment is by surgical excision.

Herniated disc can occur, particularly in the lumbar area, with pain radiation, tilting of the back, and a positive neurologic examination. An MRI will confirm the diagnosis. Treatment usually is conservative with rest, medication, bracing, and appropriate exercises, but some cases require surgery.

Rheumatoid spondylitis is rare, has a hereditary inclination, and occurs most often in adolescent males. Frequently associated with arthritis involving other joints, it presents with back pain, decreased motion, reduced chest expansion, and positive blood tests for inflammation (Erythrocyte Sedimentation Rate). Management usually is by a rheumatologist.

Hysterical back pain is diagnosed when the pain is atypical and the deformity is bizarre. The condition is common in adolescent girls. There often is a family history of back pain.

Scheuermann's disease. In adolescence the thoracic vertebrae may become wedged, producing a kyphosis (round back). This deformity most likely is due to mechanical stress superimposed on a genetically vulnerable vertebral end plate. If the deformity is severe enough to result in a cosmetic problem, it can be managed with a corrective brace. Severe kyphosis may require operative instrumentation and fusion.

Hyperlordosis (swayback) may be due to hip flexion contractures. Most cases usually resolve with growth.

Scoliosis is a lateral (to the side) curvature of the spine (Figure 9-3). This is always accompanied by rotation of the spinal column, which may be severe enough to produce a hunchback. Some curves are *functional*, meaning that they are postural in nature and will improve with growth. The body tends to compensate for a scoliotic curve by developing a secondary curve

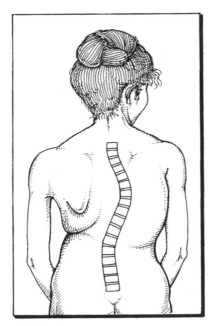

FIGURE 9-3   Scoliotic spinal curve.

above or below as well as tilting the hips and shoulders to regain an upright posture. Although initially flexible and correctable, most curves eventually will become rigid, with bony structural change leading to wedging and other permanent malformation of the vertebral bodies.

There are many notable scoliotics in history and literature, including Steinmetz, the renowned scientific electrical genius, and, as we noted, Shakespeare's Richard III, King of England, known as "crouchback." The most famous may well be Quasimodo, the hunchback of Notre Dame in Victor Hugo's novel, "Notre Dame de Paris."

The many causes of scoliosis include

- ❏ Postural (functional) related to poor posture
- ❏ Transient (related to irritation of nerve roots from a slipped disc or any other inflammation)
- ❏ Structural (this can be idiopathic [cause unknown], which comprises more than 70 percent of all cases); it often is genetic and can occur from infancy to adolescence. Girls are more affected than boys

❑ Congenital (often associated with other spinal defects)
❑ Neuromuscular—caused by diseases such as cerebral palsy, poliomyelitis, or muscular dystrophy
❑ Traumatic—secondary to injury such as fractures of the vertebrae or injuries to the thorax;
❑ Other diseases—found in various types of dwarfism, rheumatoid arthritis, osteogenesis imperfecta, or neurofibromatosis.

The treatment of scoliosis includes exercises, spinal bracing, and surgery, which consists of spinal fusion with bone grafts usually taken from the patient's pelvis or specially processed bone and/or bone substitute.

The first attempt at bone grafting was recorded by the Dutch surgeon Job Van Meekren in 1668. Since then, numerous substances have been considered to assist fracture healing and augment spinal fusion. Synthetic ceramics can be used as bone graft expanders when combined with autograft (patient's own bone). Plaster of Paris has been used as a graft material, as has demineralized bone matrix. Bone morphogenic (Gr. = structure providing) protein has been helpful in promoting spinal fusion in several animal models and holds the promise of clinical benefit in humans.

The success of electrical stimulation as an adjunct to spinal fusion has led to its increasing use over the past several decades. A variety of mechanical devices are available to augment the fusion and hold the spine in a corrected position until the graft heals and the fusion is solid. These instruments distract or compress the vertebrae or wire them to long supporting metal rods, maintaining rigid fixation and support of the corrected curve.

Scoliosis in adults can occur secondary to osteoarthritis. Surgery sometimes is necessary to relieve pain and lessen disability.

THE ADULT BACK

Low back injury is second only to the common cold as a cause of work loss in the United States. Up to 80 percent of adults will eventually experience low back pain. At any given time, about 1 percent of the work force is chronically disabled because of back problems. Upward of 100 million work days are lost each year, and billions of dollars are paid out in lawsuit awards, disability claims, and other settlements resulting from back disability. In 1996, Americans spent 53.5 million days in bed because of back pain and injury. These conditions accounted for 16.2 million physician visits and 500,000 hospitalizations, with more than 2 million days spent in hospital.

The American Academy of Orthopaedic Surgeons calculates that more than $3 billion are spent annually in the United States on the diagnosis and treatment of lumbar disc disorders. Several billion dollars more go to the physical therapists, chiropractors, acupuncturists, and a variety of other "therapists" who promote more exotic cures. The total bill for lost work time, tests, treatment, legal fees and awards, medications, and back products therefore is in excess of $80 billion a year!

Cause

What causes all this back pain? When misapplied, the long lever arm of the back can exert forces of up to 1,500 pounds per square inch on any of the vertebral bodies or, worse yet, the cushioning discs that lie between them. Sitting cannot prevent this. One of the highest measured pressures inside of the disc occurs while sitting, even higher than when standing or walking. This is why the highest risk groups for back pain are people who spend a lot of time sitting and leaning forward, such as secretaries or truck drivers.

Animals that walk on all fours, such as horses and cows, do not have to worry about back pain. Such quadripeds (four-legged animals) use a unique system of interlocking ligaments and bones in their legs that serve as a sling to suspend their body weight without strain while their muscles are completely relaxed. Because of this, a horse can stand continuously for as long as a month. However, heavy quadripeds with relatively fragile bones cannot even lie in one position for a long time because this causes muscle cramping. We bipeds gain the advantages of standing upright, which frees our arms for functional tasks and allows us to see farther than when crouched on all fours. These are positive evolutional survival features. However, we pay the price for such gifts by overloading our low backs, which have become vulnerable to low back strain and pain.

Weakened abdominal muscles fail to protect the back from the tug of abdominal organs, which can exert considerable chronic stress on both the bones and the surrounding soft tissues. Poor posture provokes the mechanical problems that initiate and perpetuate low back pain, particularly when aggravated by obesity and lack of regular exercise.

Sprains

Back sprains or strains occur when the back muscles or ligaments are stretched or torn. This usually is due to improperly performing a common activity such as bending, lifting, standing, or sitting. Holman Francis Day immortalized all this in his poem, "An old stun'wall," ... "If ye only knew the backaches in an old stun'wall." Such injury also can occur as a result of the wrenching caused by an athletic trauma or automobile accident. Practicing proper back mechanics can prevent most sprains, and the good news is that most patients with acute back pain will substantially and rapidly recover, even when their pain is severe. This prognosis holds true regardless of the treatment used or even without treatment. The bad news is that recurrences are common. Fortunately, these recurrences tend to play out much as the original incidents did, and most patients again recover quickly and spontaneously.

Consider this experiment: Bend back your index finger until it hurts. An X-ray of the finger would reveal normal bones. A biopsy would not find any notable pathology because there is none. But releasing the finger, allowing it to return to its "position of comfort," allows the pain to subside. Mechanical back pain can be considered in much the same way. The cause may be elusive, but we know which postures and activities make the back "unhappy" and which return the back to functional happiness and normal activity. This should be the goal of treatment—to restore correct posture and normal productivity.

Slipped Discs

Slipped or ruptured discs are notorious for causing pain and disability. The semisolid center of the disc may bulge or rupture through its annulus (retaining ring) to pinch the spinal nerves (Figure 9-4). This type of pain is called *sciatica* because it radi-

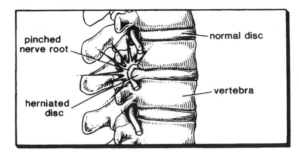

FIGURE 9-4 Herniated disc.

ates down the back of the thigh and leg in the distribution of the sciatic nerve. If it is unrelieved, permanent nerve damage can occur, resulting in numbness and muscle weakness in the leg. Most patients with slipped discs do well with nonsurgical treatment (rest, physical therapy, appropriate antiinflammatory drugs, and exercises), but approximately 10 percent require surgery. A limited approach *discectomy* (disc excision) that uses microsurgical instruments allows the surgeon to remove the herniated disc through a small incision in the lower back using an operating microscope. Because this procedure is less invasive than traditional surgery, patients can get back to their regular activities sooner.

Avoiding back injuries becomes difficult as people age. By the time most people reach the age of 40, tiny cracks in vertebral discs are the rule. It has been estimated that every fifth adult in the United States will have back pain in any given year. Most of the time these episodes are short-lived and benign. They go away in a week or two with conservative treatment. More than 90 percent of cases of acute back pain can be treated nonsurgically.

Like death and taxes, osteoarthritis cannot be avoided if you live long enough. This degenerative condition affects the discs and bones of your back in varying degree. It can narrow the disc and cause irritating spurs on the vertebral bodies, producing pain. Proper use of your back and good posture can significantly decrease the wear and tear of the degenerative arthritis of aging.

Tension and emotional problems can cause back pain. It is no coincidence that our organ language includes such phrases as "get off my back," "you're breaking my back," and the like.

Understanding the link between tension and muscle spasm can help in coping with back pain. Psychological counseling may be necessary, and presurgical psychological testing, with appropriate psychotherapy and biofeedback, can lead to improved surgical outcome.

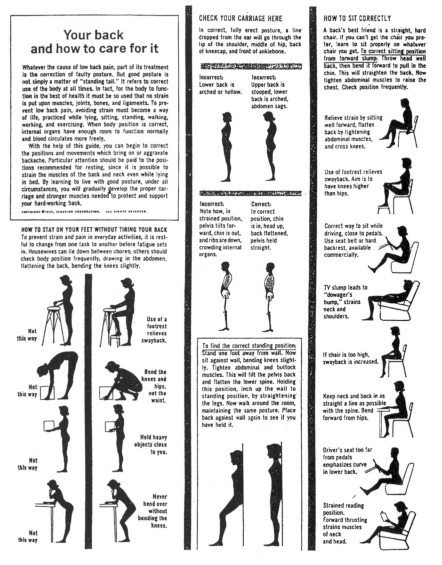

FIGURE 9-5   Your back and how to care for it (reproduced with the permission of Schering Corporation, Copyright © 1965. All rights reserved.)

Spondylolisthesis may be a problem in both adults and children. Prostate trouble or female reproductive system diseases are common causes of back pain. Tumors, particularly metastatic malignancy from such organs as the prostate, lung, thyroid, and breast, should be considered. It is important to rule out

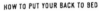

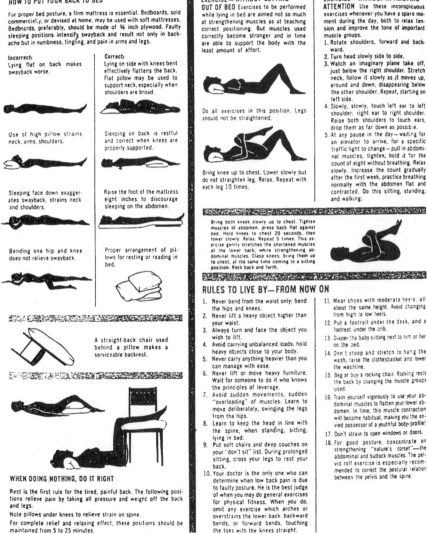

HOW TO PUT YOUR BACK TO BED

For proper bed posture, a firm mattress is essential. Bedboards, sold commercially, or devised at home, may be used with soft mattresses. Bedboards, preferably, should be made of ¾ inch plywood. Faulty sleeping positions intensify swayback and result not only in backache but in numbness, tingling, and pain in arms and legs.

Incorrect:
Lying flat on back makes swayback worse.

Correct:
Lying on side with knees bent effectively flattens the back. Flat pillow may be used to support neck, especially when shoulders are broad.

Use of high pillow strains neck, arms, shoulders.

Sleeping on back is restful and correct when knees are properly supported.

Sleeping face down exaggerates swayback, strains neck and shoulders.

Raise the foot of the mattress eight inches to discourage sleeping on the abdomen.

Bending one hip and knee does not relieve swayback.

Proper arrangement of pillows for resting or reading in bed.

A straight-back chair used behind a pillow makes a serviceable backrest.

WHEN DOING NOTHING, DO IT RIGHT

Rest is the first rule for the tired, painful back. The following positions relieve pain by taking all pressure and weight off the back and legs.

Note pillows under knees to relieve strain on spine.

For complete relief and relaxing effect, these positions should be maintained from 5 to 25 minutes.

EXERCISE—WITHOUT GETTING OUT OF BED Exercises to be performed while lying in bed are aimed not so much at strengthening muscles as at teaching correct positioning. But muscles used correctly become stronger and in time are able to support the body with the least amount of effort.

Do all exercises in this position. Legs should not be straightened.

Bring knee up to chest. Lower slowly but do not straighten leg. Relax. Repeat with each leg 10 times.

Bring both knees slowly up to chest. Tighten muscles of abdomen, press back flat against bed. Hold knees to chest 20 seconds, then lower slowly. Relax. Repeat 5 times. This exercise gently stretches the shortened muscles of the lower back, while strengthening abdominal muscles. Clasp knees, bring them up to chest, at the same time coming to a sitting position. Rock back and forth.

EXERCISE—WITHOUT ATTRACTING ATTENTION Use these inconspicuous exercises whenever you have a spare moment during the day, both to relax tension and improve the tone of important muscle groups.
1. Rotate shoulders, forward and backward.
2. Turn head slowly side to side.
3. Watch an imaginary plane take off, just below the right shoulder. Stretch neck, follow it slowly as it moves up, around and down, disappearing below the other shoulder. Repeat, starting on left side.
4. Slowly, slowly, touch left ear to left shoulder; right ear to right shoulder. Raise both shoulders to touch ears, drop them as far down as possible.
5. At any pause in the day—waiting for an elevator to arrive, for a specific traffic light to change—pull in abdominal muscles, tighten, hold it for the count of eight without breathing. Relax slowly. Increase the count gradually after the first week, practice breathing normally with the abdomen flat and contracted. Do this sitting, standing, and walking.

RULES TO LIVE BY—FROM NOW ON
1. Never bend from the waist only; bend the hips and knees.
2. Never lift a heavy object higher than your waist.
3. Always turn and face the object you wish to lift.
4. Avoid carrying unbalanced loads; hold heavy objects close to your body.
5. Never carry anything heavier than you can manage with ease.
6. Never lift or move heavy furniture. Wait for someone to do it who knows the principles of leverage.
7. Avoid sudden movements, sudden "overloading" of muscles. Learn to move deliberately, swinging the legs from the hips.
8. Learn to keep the head in line with the spine, when standing, sitting, lying in bed.
9. Put soft chairs and deep couches on your "don't sit" list. During prolonged sitting, cross your legs to rest your back.
10. Your doctor is the only one who can determine why low back pain is due to faulty posture. He is the best judge of when you may do general exercises for physical fitness. When you do, omit any exercise which arches or overstrains the lower back, backward bends, or forward bends, touching the toes with the knees straight.
11. Wear shoes with moderate heels, all about the same height. Avoid changing from high to low heels.
12. Put a footrail under the desk, and a footrest under the crib.
13. Diaper the baby sitting next to him or her on the bed.
14. Don't stoop and stretch to hang the wash; raise the clothesbasket and lower the washline.
15. Beg or buy a rocking chair. Rocking rests the back by changing the muscle groups used.
16. Train yourself vigorously to use your abdominal muscles to flatten your lower abdomen. In time, this muscle contraction will become habitual, making you the envied possessor of a youthful body-profile!
17. Don't strain to open windows or doors.
18. For good posture, concentrate on strengthening "nature's corset"—the abdominal and buttock muscles. The pelvic roll exercise is especially recommended to correct the postural relation between the pelvis and the spine.

FIGURE 9-5   (continued)

more serious causes of back pain, infrequent though they may be. Such causes occur more frequently in people younger than 20 and older than 50.

Nonmuscular causes of low back pain include vascular diseases. A deep-seated lumbar pain that does not increase with activity or decrease with rest could be due to an aortic aneurysm (weakening with thinning and ballooning of the abdominal aorta). A pain in the leg similar to sciatica is experienced in peripheral vascular disease. Neurologic causes include cysts and tumors that involve the nerve roots. Viscerogenic (Gr. = organ-generated) conditions include disease of the kidneys or pelvic viscera.

History and physical examination are the mainstay of the diagnosis of low back pain. Laboratory tests may include X-rays, CT, MRI, bone scan (to rule out tumor or infection); examination of the blood for evidence of arthritis, infection, or other contributing causes; and electrical examination of nerve and muscle function.

Treatment of Back Pain

Conservative treatment includes a brief period of bed rest, the application of heat, a pain medication, muscle relaxant, and/or NSAID, wearing a lightweight elastic lumbosacral support, and teaching good postural habits and exercises to develop proper body mechanics to keep the spine well-aligned and moving smoothly.

Exercises can help you move wisely and well by building strong, flexible muscles to support the three natural curves of your spine. Regular back exercises also help keep your spine and discs nourished and healthy, easing pain and helping to prevent injury. Back exercises fall generally into two types: flexion exercises, which are performed while you are lying on your back, and extension exercises, which are performed while you are lying on your stomach. Attention paid to tasks of daily living that involve lifting, standing, walking, driving, sitting, and sleeping can assist in avoiding back fatigue and pain. Relieving back pain during sex is possible by couples working together as understanding partners and choosing comfortable positions for intercourse.

Surgery consists of removing enough bone from the back to expose and excise a ruptured disc. Sometimes fusion of unstable vertebrae is necessary. Newer operative techniques include

A. Back lying. Man supports himself on arms and knees so very little of his weight falls on partner.

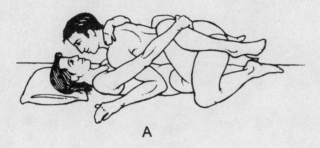

B. His back is comfortable as he maintains his natural cervical and lumbar curves with small pillows while she supports her upper body with her arms.

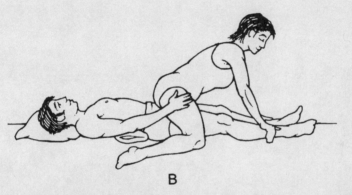

C. Stomach position may be comfortable for either partner. This position is not good for patients with neck problems.

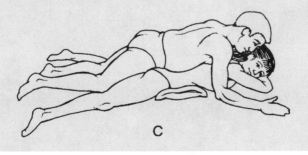

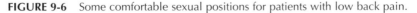

FIGURE 9-6   Some comfortable sexual positions for patients with low back pain.

D. Woman's painful back and neck are supported with small pillows or rolled towels. Man rests on his calves and heels.

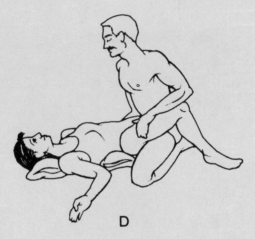

E. Kneeling. With pillows under knees, woman with back pain can easily adjust her position for maximum comfort.

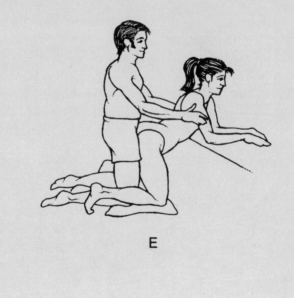

FIGURE 9-6 (continued)

F. Sitting. Back is supported with rolled towel while seated in firm chair.

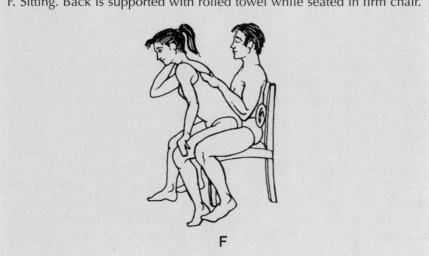

F

FIGURE 9-6   (continued)

interbody fusion, in which a cylindrical metal prop filled with bone is snugly fitted between the bodies of adjacent vertebrae. This can be performed through the abdomen using an endoscope, the same type of instrument employed to perform abdominal surgery through minimal incisions. Surgery is indicated for disc protrusions or herniations and spinal stenosis (a narrowing of the bony canal that contains the spinal cord and its nerves), arthritis, or instability of the spine leading to nerve irritation, when these do not respond to conservative treatment.

People with these conditions often are given a trial of intensive physical therapy, bed rest with traction, and oral medications (usually nonsteroidal antiinflammatory drugs, or NSAIDs). An epidural steroid injection can be prescribed, in which liquid steroid (a potent antiinflammatory medication) is injected into the area of nerve irritation, sometimes in combination with morphine. *Prolotherapy* involves injecting a solution that stiffens the soft tissue of the ligaments around the offending spinal segment. It has been claimed that this provides spinal support. Acupuncture also is becoming increasingly popular in the treatment of low back pain.

There are several absolute indications for spinal surgery. One is disc space infection, which is characterized by severe back pain and is diagnosed by an X-ray and laboratory tests that indicate inflammation (increased white blood count, elevated ESR, and the like). Infected tissue should be cleaned out of the affected disc space. Another indication for surgery is the *cauda equina syndrome*. This is due to acute pressure on the nerves at the termination of the spinal cord or on the cord itself. A high herniated lumbar disc, among other things, can cause this. The patient with a cauda equina syndrome is in severe pain and has sensory loss in a saddle distribution about the buttocks. The real tip-off is difficulty urinating and/or having a bowel movement. There is rapid and progressive loss of motor and sensory function in the legs. A *myelogram*, a procedure in which X-rays are taken after an absorbable radiopaque dye is injected into the spinal fluid, will reveal complete blockage at the level of disc herniation. Cauda equina syndrome is a surgical emergency requiring immediate operative relief of pressure on the spine or its nerves.

Chemonucleolysis entails injecting directly into the disc an enzyme similar to the papaya extract used in meat tenderizer. This dissolves a portion of the disc, allowing the remainder to shrink and retract and thus taking pressure off the nerve. This procedure carries some risk (particularly if you are one of the unlucky few who happen to be allergic to the enzyme) and requires considerable skill to perform.

Electrocoagulation is yet another technique used to shrink the disc. It can be done after a discogram is performed. This is an X-ray that localizes the offending disc(s) by injecting absorbable radiopaque dye into the disc(s), reproducing the pain related to disc herniation and revealing X-ray evidence of disc degeneration.

Sacroiliac joint dysfunction presents with an atypical pattern of back pain but no intraspinal pathology, such as spinal stenosis or a herniated disc. Physical therapy, NSAIDs, and a sacroiliac belt usually alleviate disabling symptoms. Surgery to fuse the joint is safe and effective in appropriately chosen patients.

Transcutaneous electrical nerve stimulation (TENS) is often used for chronic low back pain, as are manipulation and injection of painful "trigger points" with local anesthetic and a corticosteroid medication or direct injection of the facet joints of the vertebrae.

Many patients suffer from such painful "trigger points" associated with myofascial pain disorders such as fibromyalgia. Treatment is with medications and the injection of these trigger points with Novocain and sometimes a steroid drug. Forceful pressure to the painful point also will give relief. An easy way to provide pressure to hard-to-reach areas of the back is to place a used tennis ball (because it is more pliable than a new one) in a long sock. Stand with your back against a wall and lower the ball over your shoulders to the area of the trigger point. Now, lean back against the ball for a full minute. The pain will first increase, but then it should ease.

Try to remember that an ounce of prevention is worth a pound of cure in the prevention and treatment of low back pain. You can keep your back fit by maintaining good posture and following a well-balanced program of exercise, as well as avoiding back strain. Try to keep your low back straight, avoiding swayback, and always lift with your legs, not with your back. Sleeping and sitting habits are important. You should sit in a firm chair that supports your back and should sleep on a level, firm mattress.

If you take some basic precautions and make some changes now, you can help prevent serious back problems later. Severe, persistent, or recurrent back pain should be reported to your doctor, especially if you experience numbness and/or pain down either leg. Unexplained weight loss, fever, difficulty with bowel or bladder function, a history of injury or osteoporosis, vascular disease, or steroid or intravenous drug use are all "red flags" for more serious disease. Take charge of your back and you will stay out of trouble.

You can get more information on back care on the Internet. Here are some recommended sites (taken from *Back Pain on the Net—The Journal of Musculoskeletal Medicine*, March, 2000, pp. 130–140).

INTERNET ADDRESSES OF RECOMMENDED SITES FOR BACK CARE INFORMATION

Home Pages

American Academy of Pain Management
    www.aapainmanage.org/index.html

The Back Letter
    news.medscape.com/LWW/BL/public/BL-journal.html

Journal of the Southern Orthopaedic Association
    www.sma.org/soa/jsoa.htm

Medscape Orthopaedics & Sports Medicine
    orthopedics. medscape.com/Medscape/
    OrthoSportsMed/journal/public/mos.journal.html

National Institutes of Health
    www.nih.gov

San Francisco Spine Institute
    www.spinecare.com

Spine-health.com
    www.spine-health.com/index1.html

Texas Back Institute
    www.texasback.com

University of Washington Bone and Joint Sources
    www.orthop.washington.edu

Useful Patient Information

Back Pain Mini Information Sheet
    www.ninds.nih.gov/patients/disorder/back pain/
    backpain.htm

"Chronic Pain: Hope Through Research"
    www.ninds.nih.gov/patients/disorder/chrpain/
    chronic-pain.htm

"Do I Need an MRI?"
    www.spine-health.com/fe/mri/m01.html

Find a Pain Management Program
    www.aapainmanage.org/aapm/ppdsrcht.html

Getting Your Spine in Shape
    www.texasback.com/html/
    getting_your_spine_in_shape.html

"Golf and Low Back Pain"
    www.spine-health.com/fe/golf/g01.html

Treatment Options
www.texasback.com/html/treatment_options.html

"What is Physiatry?"
www.spine-health.com/fe/physi/p01.html

CASE REPORT—Low Back Pain

Arnold K. is a 45-year-old office worker who leads a sedentary life. His only exercise is taking neighborhood walks with his wife and an occasional swim in the summer. While shaving one morning, Arnold bent over and experienced severe low back pain that radiated down the back of his legs to his knees. He could not bend, and his wife had to help him dress so he could get to work. The pain was so excruciating that he left work early, went home, and went directly to bed. Arnold took an over-the-counter pain medication and stayed in bed with a heating pad on his back. This helped a little, but he was still stiff and in pain the next morning, so his wife drove him to their doctor.

The doctor found that Arnold had a severe muscle spasm in his low back. His neurologic examination was normal, and an X-ray of the back was negative for arthritis or other pathology. Because Arnold had no history of serious risk factors or comorbidities (other significant diseases), the doctor did not order further tests at the time of the initial visit and elected to treat Arnold conservatively. He was advised to rest at home for a day or two, using a firm sleeping surface. Arnold was instructed in proper back care, including bending from the knees, not the back, tightening the abdomen and flattening the back, and back protective techniques for reaching and lifting. A light elastic back support was provided and an NSAID was prescribed. Arnold was told to use moist heat on his back.

After several days of rest, Arnold felt well enough to return to work part-time. A program of rehabilitative exercises was started, and he was advised to reduce his weight by 15 pounds. The doctor told Arnold to join a local health club where he could work out in a back reconditioning program and swim several times a week. By following this program, Arnold generally feels much better and has avoided recurrence of his low back pain.

QUESTIONS AND ANSWERS—THE SPINE

Q: How do I know when my back is bad enough to consult my doctor?

A: It is certainly time to see your doctor if:

❑ The pain is severe enough to keep you up at night and away from work.

❑ You have tried home remedies for a few days and you are not getting better or are getting worse.

❑ You have noticed weakness in your legs or have any difficulty urinating or moving your bowels.

❑ You have pain or numbness radiating into your legs.

If you have risk factors for vascular disease (high cholesterol, smoking, and the like), are using steroids, have a history of osteoporosis, cancer, or a substantial trauma, unexplained weight loss, or no matter how hard you try, you cannot find a comfortable position, you may have a more serious illness that requires immediate medical attention.

Q: If, as Shakespeare notes regarding Falstaf, "the belly robs the back," what is the best exercise for strengthening the abdominal muscles?

A: Partial sit-ups or abdominal curls are the best exercises for strengthening the muscles of the abdomen. It is important to perform these exercises with the knees bent so the back is not strained. Partial sit-ups are done with the arms behind the head, abdominal curls with the arms crossed over the stomach. During both exercises the pelvis should be tilted, pressing the small of the back into the supporting surface. For a sit-up, the torso should be brought almost to the sitting position; for a curl-up, the head and shoulders should be curled up until the shoulder blades have cleared the floor and the position held for a moment. You should start with as many repetitions as can be easily performed, gradually increasing the exercise until a maximum of 50 to 100 can be accomplished during one exercise period.

Q: Should everyone sleep on an extra firm mattress?

A: Most people, particularly those who have a back problem, are more comfortable on an extra firm mattress.

However, a few people seem to prefer a softer mattress or even a waterbed. If you are one of these, by all means continue to use the type of mattress that provides the most comfort.

Q: Are exercises that *flex* the back (bend it forward) better than exercises that *extend* the back (bend it backward)?

A: Exercises that flex the back are called Williams exercises. These are excellent for limbering up the low back. Exercises that extend the back are called Mackenzie exercises. These help to strengthen the low back and are prescribed for patients with "disc pain."

Flexion exercises are performed while lying on your back and bending your knees up to your body. This flattens your back.

Extension exercises involve lying on your stomach and arching your back by pressing up with your arms. People also test various motions to see which positions can "centralize" their pain, causing it to retreat toward the midline. Both exercises are valuable in treating low back pain. All exercises should be supervised by a knowledgeable therapist.

Q: Are there any new "cutting edge" treatments for low back pain?

A: A great deal of research is being conducted into new treatments for low back pain. One procedure is *intradiscal electrothermal therapy* (IDET). This is an outpatient procedure that is used to treat bulging or degenerated lumbar discs. It involves placing, under direct visual control with fluoroscopy, a thin catheter into the center of the disc. Thermal energy (heat) is then applied to contract and thicken the collagen of the annulus fibrosus. Heating the collagen does two things. It causes it to contract and tighten, and the nociceptors (pain nerve fibers) in the disc are destroyed. Early studies show a reduction of disc pain in 70 to 80 percent of patients.

Another procedure is *kyphoplasty*. This is indicated for the treatment of osteoporotic vertebral compression fractures. Through a very small skin incision (stab wound) an inflatable balloon is threaded under fluoroscopy into the center of the fractured vertebra. The balloon is inflated and the vertebral compression fracture is realigned. Then the center of the vertebra is filled with bone cement in an effort to restore normal vertebral height and alignment. The safety and effectiveness of this procedure are currently being evaluated.

Q: Does smoking impair healing in bone and soft tissues?

A: Several well-controlled studies have indicated that cigarette smoking has a detrimental effect on the healing of soft tissues and bone. Cigarettes contain toxic compounds that interfere with normal tissue metabolism, and nicotine may affect the ingrowth of blood vessels into healing bone. Patients undergoing orthopaedic procedures such as spinal fusion, fusion in the foot, or repair of the rotator cuff of the shoulder are at a significantly increased risk of having a poor result from their surgical procedure than those who are nonsmokers or who have discontinued smoking before surgery.

Q: What is spinal stenosis?

A: Spinal stenosis is a form of sciatica (pain referred down the sciatic nerve) resulting from narrowing of the lumbar spinal canal, causing pressure on the nerve roots or, rarely, the spinal cord itself. Pain in the legs can be intermittent on activity, mimicking vascular disease such as arteriosclerosis. Spinal stenosis occurs in middle-aged or elderly patients. The most common cause is osteoarthritis of the spine. There is pain in the buttocks, thighs, or calves on walking, running, or climbing stairs. The pain is not relieved by standing still but by flexing the back (bending forward) or sitting. Walking up hills is less painful than walking down, because the back is flexed. Severity of the pain is relieved by rest. Numbness in the legs may occur. Decompressive laminectomies (removing bony pressure on the sciatic spinal nerve roots) at several levels may be required if conservative measures such as improved posture, bracing, NSAIDs, weight loss, and abdominal muscle strengthening fail to provide relief.

Now let's work our way down the arm, starting with the shoulder.

10

The Shoulder

"Behind ye yer shoulders stick out like two boulders;
Yer shins are as thin as a pair of pen-holders!"
Robert W. Chambers
The Recruit

The shoulder is actually a complex of four joints. What most people think about when they refer to the shoulder is the *glenohumeral joint*, the ball-and-socket joint between the upper arm-bone and the scapula (shoulder blade), but the scapula articulates (joins) with the rib cage to form the *scapulothoracic joint* and with the *clavicle* (collarbone) to form the *acromioclavicular joint*. Finally, the clavicle articulates with the sternum (breast plate), shaping the sternoclavicular joint. These joints all participate in shoulder movements. Because there are so many of them, and because the shoulder sacrifices stability for mobility so we can perform wonderful athletic tasks like turning a cartwheel or pitching a no-hit baseball game, the shoulder sustains more injuries than any other part of the upper extremity. The ultimate function of the shoulder complex is to facilitate movement of the arm to ensure appropriate placing of the hand for effective use. The shoulder joints are interdependent yet move in concert with each other. It therefore follows that a problem with one of the joints would affect the function of the others, as indeed it does.

ANATOMY

The round ball at the top of the humerus (upper arm bone) is held in the shallow *glenoid* (shoulder socket) by the tendons of a

165

group of muscles originating from the front and back of the scapula (Greek—I dig = a spade, which it looks like) articulates with the clavicle (Latin—clavis = a key, because its shape resembles that of a key). These soft tissue structures fuse to form the *rotator cuff*, which, along with the capsule of the joint, hold the shoulder in place as well as move it. As in the hip, the socket is deepened by a soft tissue rim called the glenoid labrum (Greek = socket, Latin = lip) (Figure 10-1).

INJURIES

The lateral extension of the spine of the scapula that projects over the shoulder joint to form the highest point of the shoulder is called the *acromion* (Greek—acro = top, omos = shoulder). This is where the scapula articulates with the clavicle. Problems with this joint are fairly common in athletes.

The space between the acromion and the rotator cuff contains a *bursa*. This bursa or the underlying cuff can become inflamed because of impingement between the underside of the acromion and the cuff during vigorous shoulder movement.

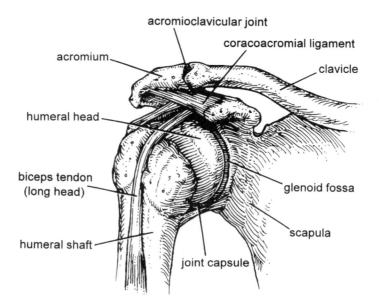

FIGURE 10-1   Anatomy of your shoulder.

Increased laxity of ligaments makes women more susceptible to shoulder impingement, especially female athletes whose activity requires repeated overhead arm movements, such as swimming (particularly with the crawl or butterfly stroke) or racquet sports.

The aim of treatment is to detect the condition early and prevent progression to more serious injury. The shoulder should be rested, and ice and ultrasound should be used to decrease pain and swelling. An injection of corticosteroid medication into the subacromial space occasionally is indicated. An NSAID is prescribed to reduce inflammation, and stretching and strengthening exercises should be performed as pain permits. Surgery, which can be accomplished through an arthroscope, consists of a decompression procedure that enlarges the space by removing offending soft tissue and bone.

Rotator cuff tears can develop as a result of repeated impingement or can occur suddenly because of a fall on an outstretched hand. A small or partial tear may heal with rest, but a full thickness rotator cuff tear calls for surgical repair, which may require either a highly technical arthroscopic procedure or open surgical repair.

Calcification in the rotator cuff can occur as a response to injury. The calcific mass may resemble a milky emulsion, may have a thick toothpaste-like consistency, or may be granular and gritty. Because it is so painful, it has been called a "sterile boil" of the shoulder. Treatment consists of removal by needling and aspiration or opening the deposit and scraping out the offending calcium.

Adhesive capsulitis or "frozen shoulder" is a condition in which there is spontaneous onset of shoulder pain followed by increasingly severe restriction of shoulder motion. This condition occurs in both men and women, usually between the ages of 40 to 60 years. The nondominant shoulder seems to be affected more often than the dominant. Frozen shoulder is common in patients with arthritis of the neck, diabetes, and after heart attacks. There appears to be a suggestion of an inflammatory process, and the joint capsule becomes scarred and stuck to surrounding structures.

In its early stages, adhesive capsulitis can be treated with vigorous exercise, electrical stimulation, and passive (stretching) mobilization of the shoulder. Manipulation of the shoulder

A. Elevation. Raising hand as far as possible, grasp a stable surface. Keep your arm straight and lower your body by bending knees. You will feel your shoulder stretching.

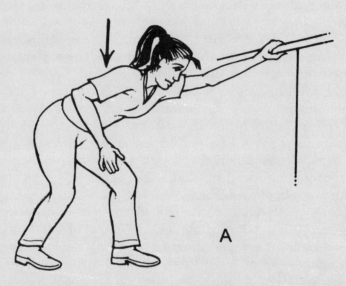

B. External rotation (turning out). Standing in a doorway, grasp the door jamb with the hand on the side of the stiff shoulder. With your other hand, hold the elbow on the stiff side firmly against your body. Now, rotate your body away from the door jamb. You will feel your shoulder stretching.

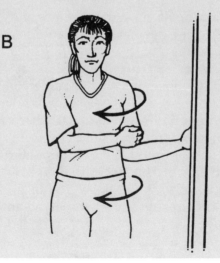

FIGURE 10-2   Shoulder exercises to restore flexibility.

C. Internal rotation (turning in). Move the arm of your stiff shoulder toward the middle of your back with your palm facing out. Use your other hand to push your arm up until you feel the stretch in your shoulder.

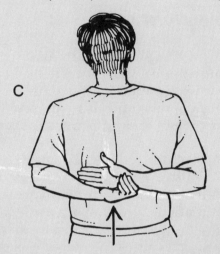

D. Adduction (reaching across). Place the hand from the stiff side over the opposite shoulder. Try to raise your elbow as close to shoulder height as you can. Use your other hand to push the raised elbow toward the opposite shoulder. You will feel a stretch in the painful shoulder.

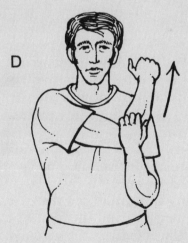

General note: These four exercises are excellent for frozen shoulder or rehabilitation after shoulder injury. They should be performed daily in sets of 6–12 repetitions.

FIGURE 10-2   (continued)

under anesthesia or arthroscopic release of the tight capsule can be carried out if conservative measures fail.

SHOULDER DISLOCATION

Most dislocations of the shoulder are anterior (to the front), although occasionally a posterior (to the back) dislocation can occur. There are several methods for manually reducing a dislocated shoulder. Muscle relaxation is necessary, and the operator must be careful not to use undue force or the shoulder will break in the attempt.

Every time a shoulder dislocates, the soft tissue structures are injured, the shoulder capsule is stretched, and it becomes increasingly easy for the shoulder to dislocate again. After several recurrent dislocations, the shoulder may spontaneously dislocate while the patient is turning during sleep. There are a number of surgical procedures, including capsular reefing and repair, reattachment of a torn labrum, and bone wedges to block dislocation, for the operative treatment of recurrent dislocation of the shoulder.

Fracture of the head and neck of the humerus is a serious injury that occurs in older people. It is important to obtain anatomic reduction in order to avoid the complication of late-onset traumatic arthritis. Because early motion is desirable to avoid adhesions and stiffness, open reduction with internal metallic fixation is often the procedure of choice.

An irritation of the bony growth zone (*epiphysis*) of children who participate in Little League baseball is called *Little League shoulder*. Traction of the muscles about the shoulder results in irritation of the growth zone of the upper humerus. X-rays may reveal bony reaction to the trauma. The disorder is treated with rest and leaves no residual.

Shoulder pointer is an injury to the tip of the shoulder from a direct blow. The muscles and the joint at the end of the clavicle (collarbone) at the shoulder (the acromioclavicular joint) are injured. The damage usually heals in short order with rest, ice, and a nonsteroidal antiinflammatory drug (NSAID).

Shoulder separation refers to a partial or complete dislocation of the clavicle where it joins the shoulder at the *acromioclavicular joint*. When minor, such an injury can be treated with

PENDULUM EXERCISES
FOR SHOULDER MOBILIZATION

THE FOLLOWING EXERCISES ARE PERFORMED WHILE STANDING AND LEANING FORWARD AT THE WAIST. THE UPPER BODY SHOULD BE HORIZONTAL TO THE FLOOR. HOLD ON TO A STATIONARY OBJECT WITH THE UNAFFECTED ARM FOR SUPPORT. THE AFFECTED ARM SHOULD BE COMPLETELY RELAXED AND SHOULD HANG LOOSELY TOWARD THE FLOOR. TO INCREASE COMFORT AND RELAXATION A TWO-POUND WEIGHT MAY BE HELD IN THE HAND ON THE AFFECTED SIDE WHILE DOING THE EXERCISE.

PENDULUM EXERCISE #1

EXTEND THE AFFECTED ARM TOWARD THE FLOOR AND SWING IT LIKE A PENDULUM IN GRADUALLY INCREASING CIRCLES. THEN GRADUALLY DECREASE THE SIZE OF THE CIRCLES AND LET THE ARM COME TO A COMPLETE STOP. MAKE THE CIRCLES FIRST CLOCKWISE AND THEN COUNTER-CLOCKWISE.

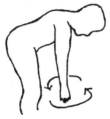

PENDULUM EXERCISE #2

IN SAME MANNER AS IN EXERCISE #1, SWING YOUR ARM; ONLY THIS TIME SWING IT FORWARD AND BACKWARD. GRADUALLY INCREASE THE SIZE OF THE SWINGS AND THEN GRADUALLY DECREASE THE SWINGS.

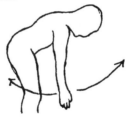

PENDULUM EXERCISE #3

SWING YOUR ARM FROM SIDE TO SIDE: FIRST ACROSS IN FRONT OF YOUR BODY AND THEN OUT TO THE SIDE.

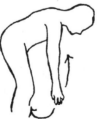

FIGURE 10-3   Pendulum exercises for maintaining or restoring shoulder motion.

rest. However, a complete separation in the dominant shoulder of an athlete whose sport requires throwing (commonly a football quarterback) often will require surgical repair. With complete dislocation, except for an unsightly bump on the shoulder, most individuals have no pain or serious disability. The dislocation can be treated by support in a sling for three to six weeks until healing is complete. If the deformity is too unsightly or if painful arthritis occurs in the joint after injury, a simple operation to remove a small portion of the clavicle at the shoulder can be performed at a later date.

Slipping shoulder is due to weakness and stretching of the shoulder capsule, which permits the joint to slip yet not fully dislocate. Symptoms include pain, weakness, and apprehension, particularly when the arm is rotated up and out. Sometimes appropriate exercises can strengthen the muscles of the shoulder and prevent slipping. When this fails, a surgical procedure is available to tighten the stretched structures and restore stability to the shoulder. *Thermal capsular shift*, which uses heat to shrink and tighten the tissues that support the shoulder, is a new technique available for selected cases of shoulder instability.

ARTHRITIS

Painful degeneration of the shoulder is common in people with rheumatoid arthritis. Primary shoulder osteoarthritis is uncommon but can occur following trauma to the shoulder. Severe arthritic pain in the shoulder that is unrelieved by conservative measures such as physiotherapy and intraarticular steroid injections can be treated by total shoulder replacement. In this procedure, the articular surface of the humeral head is removed and a metal humeral prosthesis similar to the femoral component of a total hip replacement is inserted down the shaft of the humerus. The glenoid may or may not be replaced. The glenoid component (like the acetabular moiety in hip replacement) is either made entirely of plastic or metal-backed, depending on its design. The components can be inserted with or without bone cement.

CASE REPORT—The Shoulder

Todd S. was an active 52-year-old executive. He had been an athlete in high school and attended college on a football scholarship. He was a member of a health club, where he ran and worked out several times a week. After an unusually vigorous workout session that included over-head weight lifting, Todd began to experience pain in his right (dominant) shoulder. He applied moist heat and took a few over-the-counter pain pills, but the discomfort persisted. The pain was worse when he attempted to reach or lift his arm to the side. When his condition did not improve after several weeks of home care, Todd's wife became concerned and urged him to see their doctor, which he did.

An X-ray was negative, but physical examination revealed that Todd's right shoulder was tender in the front and side. It also was weaker than the left shoulder, whereas it should have been as strong or even stronger because Todd was right-handed. The muscles of the shoulder had atrophied (shrunk). Todd was referred to an orthopaedic surgeon, who made a diagnosis of *impingement syndrome*. The shoulder was injected with a steroid solution, and an NSAID was prescribed. Todd began physical therapy treatments that included ultrasound, massage, and pendulum exercises to keep the shoulder from stiffening. Todd's shoulder improved, but his pain did not entirely resolve. Therefore, an MRI was ordered. The MRI showed significant wear in the tendons of the rotator cuff with partial tearing. An arthroscopic repair was performed, and after an appropriate period of rehabilitation, which included graded exercises, Todd was symptom-free and able to return to recreational athletics, although he was cautioned to avoid heavy overhead lifting.

QUESTIONS AND ANSWERS—THE SHOULDER

Q: What is a "stinger?"

A: Stretching of the nerves that enter the arm from the neck (the brachial plexus) is unique to the sport of American football. Such an injury is called a "stinger" or "burner." It results from a sudden and violent depression of the shoulder with stretching of the neck in the opposite direction. This often occurs when ramming the head in tackling or blocking. The "stinger" is characterized by sudden pain in the neck that radiates to the hand. The pain is burning in nature, and transient weakness may occur. Treatment usually is unnecessary. However, if symptoms persist for more than a few minutes, a more serious injury, even a fracture in the neck, should be ruled out before the athlete is allowed to return to play.

Q: Is fusion of the shoulder ever necessary? Is it a disabling operation?

A: Any loss of joint movement can be disabling, particularly if remaining movement is painful. However, there are some conditions for which shoulder *arthrodesis* (fusion) is indicated. These include poliomyelitis or other neuromuscular conditions or injuries that leave the patient with a paralyzed, functionless shoulder. If the rest of the arm is working, stabilizing the shoulder should enable the patient to use his hand for grooming, feeding, and other tasks of daily living. Some other indications for shoulder fusion include destruction and/or severe pain related to infection, advanced arthritis, or serious trauma. The shoulder should be fused in a position of maximal function, slightly forward and outward at the joint, the so-called "salute" position.

Q: What is congenital pseudarthrosis of the clavicle?

A: This is a rare defect of uncertain cause. It usually occurs on the right side and consists of a defect in the middle part of the clavicle. The term *pseudarthrosis* means false (pseudo) joint (arthrosis). It can produce narrowing and weakness of the shoulder as well as an unsightly lump at the middle of the clavicle. The major disability is cosmetic. Surgery, which is best undertaken in early childhood, is the preferred treatment. It consists of excision of the pseudarthrosis, bone grafting, and fixation with a plate and screws.

Q: Why is osteoarthritis relatively uncommon in the shoulder?

A: Osteoarthritis is a degenerative condition that occurs mostly in weight-bearing joints such as the hips and knees, which are subjected to repeated loading stress and strain. However, people who chronically overload and abuse their shoulders, even through the prolonged use of a cane, can develop osteoarthritis in their shoulders.

Q: What is habitual shoulder subluxation?

A: Very loose-jointed adolescents can voluntarily sublux or even dislocate one or both shoulders. Management of this condition is difficult because there usually is a strong psychological element that perpetuates the practice. Avoiding voluntary displacement, strengthening exercises, and psychological counseling are appropriate. Resolution usually occurs with time if the child can find more appropriate methods of getting attention. Operations should be avoided.

Q: What is obstetrical palsy?

A: Obstetrical palsy results from an injury to the nerves that travel to the arm (the brachial plexus) that occurs during delivery. The extent of loss of function in the arm is determined by the level of the injury. Improved obstetrical practice has decreased the incidence of these injuries. Approximately 75 percent spontaneously resolve during the first year of life. Early repair of the damaged nerves has been attempted by some adventuresome surgeons. For unresolved weakness about the shoulder and arm, tendon transfers and bony operations are available later during childhood.

Our shoulders function to move our elbows, which move our wrists, which move our hands. So let's now go down and talk about the joint next in line, the elbow.

11

The Elbow

My elbow itchid! I thought there would a scab follow.
William Shakespeare
Much Ado About Nothing, *III, III, 106*

The elbow is more than a simple hinge joint. True, you can bend your elbow up as much as 145° with a hingelike motion. But the elbow also rotates. The bones and muscles of your elbow allow you to supinate (turn your hand palm-up) and pronate (turn your hand palm-down). All of these functions are made possible by the three bones that meet to form the elbow joint, the *humerus* (upper arm bone) and the *radius* and the *ulna* (bones of the forearm). The hinge joint consists of the *humeroulnar* and *humeroradial* joints, at which flexion (bending) and extension (straightening) take place. Pronation and supination occur in the radioulnar joint, facilitated by the humeroradial joint.

The bump you feel at the back of the elbow is the *olecranon* (Greek = point of the elbow) process of the ulna (Latin = arm). The bumps you feel on each side of your elbow are epicondyles (bony knobs of the humerus), which serve as points of attachment for muscles. A bursa (Latin = purse) pads the tip of the elbow at the olecranon, permitting your skin to slide over the bone.

Most of the long muscles that move the hand are attached at the elbow. The *extensor-supinator* muscles that originate from the outside of the elbow supinate (from the Latin supinus = lying on the back) the forearm, bringing the palm up as in prayer and allowing you to eat or use a screwdriver. The *flexor-*

pronator muscles that originate from the inside of the elbow pronate the forearm, bringing the palm down (from the Latin pronare = to turn face downard), allowing you to write or close a doorknob.

The important *ulnar nerve* lies close to the surface of the elbow, running through a groove along the inside of the joint to provide motor power to the forearm and hand as well as sensation to the last two fingers. Strong ligaments connect the bones of the elbow to hold them in place (Figure 11-1).

ELBOW INJURIES

The many bones and soft tissues of your elbow play an important part in providing a complete range of motion for your arms and hands. Elbow injuries can be painful enough to prevent you from using your wrist and hand.

Early diagnosis can help you recover more quickly and completely from an elbow condition. Your doctor will take a history and ask you what particular activities cause pain in your elbow and whether you have suffered an elbow injury before. A physi-

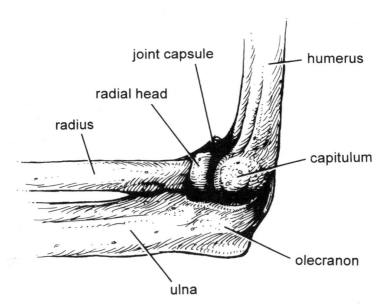

FIGURE 11-1   Anatomy of your elbow.

cal examination will be performed, including measurement of range of motion and assessment of strength. Diagnostic tests may include X-rays or other imaging techniques as well as an aspiration to remove fluid from the joint for evaluation. Blood tests are used to check for arthritis or infection. Diagnostic arthroscopy occasionally is required.

Common conditions that affect the elbow include lateral and medial epicondylitis. *Lateral epicondylitis* ("tennis elbow") usually is due to a frayed or inflamed elbow tendon and involves the outer elbow. An improper backhand stroke is almost always the cause of tennis elbow in tennis players. Chris Evert-Lloyd, Bjorn Borg, Jimmy Conners, and others, in popularizing the two-handed backhand, have done much to decrease the incidence of tennis elbow. However, the condition also occurs in anyone engaging in any activity that requires twisting the wrist with the elbow straight. Factory workers, mechanics, and homemakers are prone to this annoying injury.

Treatment is first to stop—or at least modify—the offending activity. Tennis players should play their backhand with elbow and wrist rigid. The racquet should be large and made of metal alloy or other springy composite material designed to reduce elbow stress on ball contact. Increasing the grip size of the racquet with padding sometimes can help. A strap wrapped just below the elbow will block the force generated by the inflamed elbow tendon (usually that of the extensor carpi radialis brevis muscle), granting some relief during play. Icing and aspirin or other NSAIDs are prescribed, and local injections of steroids can alleviate pain. Acupuncture sometimes helps. Forearm strengthening exercises such as wrist curls can prevent recurrences. Resistant cases require surgery to release the tendon at its origin.

When the inside of the elbow is involved, the condition is called *medial epicondylitis* ('golfer's elbow"). Golfer's elbow is much less common than tennis elbow and is not as disabling. Treatment is similar to that for tennis elbow.

Improper use of the elbow in reaching or gripping at work can cause epicondylitis as the result of a repetitive strain syndrome. Workplace modifications are an important part of any treatment program.

Physical therapy, especially the use of ultrasound, a form of deep heat produced by sonic vibrations, sometimes is prescribed. Special elbow exercises designed to improve and maintain

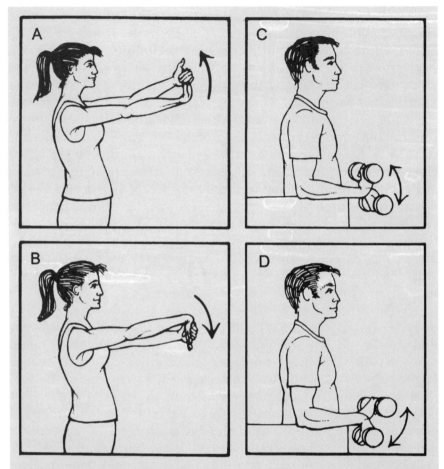

Stretching (a and b): Extend arm and hold wrist firmly back for slow count of six. Repeat six times.

Strengthening (c and d): Wrist curls and reverse wrist curls can be performed with a one or two pound dumbbell or or light weight. Perform 12–24 repetitions as illustrated.

FIGURE 11-2   Stretching and strengthening exercises for tennis elbow.

strength in the elbow muscles are important for rehabilitation. Warm-up and cool-down stretches before and after play can help prevent injury and improve both your tennis game and your golf game.

"Little League elbow" is caused by the repetitive act of throwing, which places great stress on the elbow, and occurs par-

ticularly in pitchers. Because their bony structures are immature, children are subject to having chips of bone torn off (*avulsion fractures*), developing an inflammation of the growing parts
of the bone (osteochondritis), having loose cartilage in the joint
(joint mice), and a variety of other bony and soft tissue injuries.

The elbow is painful and stiff. Symptoms may be either
acute or chronic in nature. Examination reveals a restricted
range of motion, and an X-ray may show bony injury and/or
effusion (fluid) in the joint. For the Little Leaguer, treatment
usually is conservative, consisting of rest and eliminating the
offending activity. Some of these injuries require months of inactivity in order to heal. In the case of a loose body, surgical
removal can be performed, usually through an arthroscope.

The best treatment for Little League elbow is prevention. In
order to protect the elbow, no more than five to six innings of
baseball should be pitched each week, and at least four to five
days off are needed between games.

SPRAINS

Sprains of the ligaments that support the elbow (collateral ligaments) are not as common or as severe as those of the knee. This
is because the elbow is a non–weight-bearing joint. Treatment
usually is conservative with a plaster splint, rest in a sling,
icing, and an NSAID. Surgical repair is necessary if complete
rupture has occurred.

Because we often lean on our elbows and they can easily be
bumped, bursitis of the olecranon bursa is common. A painful
swelling results. Your doctor may aspirate excess fluid and inject
cortisone into the bursa to decrease inflammation. Recurrent or
chronic bursitis will require resection of the olecranon bursa.

When you hit your "funny bone," you have actually hit your
ulnar nerve. *Neuritis* (nerve inflammation) can occur if pressure is
applied to the nerve over a long period of time. Just repeatedly
leaning heavily on your elbow can do this. With ulnar neuritis you
will feel tingling and numbness in your last two fingers and may
experience some weakness of these digits. As the nerve is pressed
between skin and bone along the inside of your elbow, the joint
may begin to ache. Conservative treatment consists of avoiding
leaning on the elbow (or wearing an elbow pad) as well as a brief

course of antiinflammatory or analgesic drugs. Occasionally surgery (transposition of the ulnar nerve from its groove) is necessary.

DISLOCATION

The elbow can be dislocated by falling on an outstretched hand.
With proper relaxation of the patient it is usually reduced without difficulty and then held in a splint or sling. Early motion is
encouraged because after injury the elbow can stiffen faster
than any other joint in the body.

FRACTURES

Any bone about the elbow can be broken. Fractures into the
joint are serious because they often cause arthritis and limit
motion. Common fractures include fracture of the head of the
radius. The radial head jams against the capitellum (Latin = little head) of the humerus and is either cracked or completely broken with displacement of the fragments. With a simple crack,
early motion is encouraged. With a more severe fracture, the
radial head can be excised. However, this is never done in a
child before growth is complete because the structure of the
forearm would be compromised.

Fractures of the olecranon are also common. They are due
to a direct blow to the tip of the elbow. Treatment usually is surgical. The fracture pieces are wired or screwed together, and
early movement is encouraged. Fractures of the humerus at the
elbow also can occur and often require surgery. Arthroscopy is
sometimes used to help a surgeon see and remove fragments of
loose bone from the joint. Fixation by pins, by screws, or by
wires are surgical options. Tension band wiring, which com-
presses the fracture fragments and expedites union, is a good
surgical technique for treating an olecranon fracture.

ARTHRITIS

Severe arthritis of the elbow is common in people with rheumatoid arthritis. Once there is bony destruction of the joint accom-

panied by pain, a total elbow replacement can be performed. The aim of this operation is to relieve pain, not so much to improve range of motion. Although a prosthesis for the radial head is available, simple excision of the radial head in the case of advanced arthritis usually is enough to relieve pain and maintain motion.

COMPARTMENT SYNDROME

Because the muscles of the upper extremity are enclosed in thick unyielding fascial coverings or envelopes, they are vulnerable to damage from swelling or any other cause of increased pressure. Soft tissue or bony injury to the forearm as well as the elbow can cause such a *compartment syndrome* (similar to that which can occur in the calf) If the increased pressure is not detected early and the compartment is not surgically decompressed, a *Volkmann's ischemic contracture* can result. This condition is due to lack of blood supply to the muscles of the forearm, which occurs because of the increased pressure. It also can occur when the brachial artery is damaged at the elbow as a result of a dislocation or fracture. Volkmann's ischemic contracture results in flexion deformity of the wrist and fingers, caused by scarring and subsequent contracture of the muscles of the forearm. It is a serious disability that is not easily remedied by therapy and/or surgery.

CASE REPORT—The Elbow

Stanley B., 12 years old, was the star pitcher for his Little League team. Stanley's dreams of a career in professional baseball were encouraged by his parents, who were justifiably proud of his many trophies. Stanley's coach was equally enthusiastic as his team, the "Marionville Musketeers," were headed for their first state title under Stanley's pitching, bolstered by the .350 batting averages of several preteen sluggers. One day after a close win with Stanley pitching nine innings, Stanley complained of pain in his elbow. After the game, he iced the elbow and took some aspirin. However, the pain persisted and the elbow was swollen and markedly tender. Examination by the school physician

continued on next page

---

revealed a restricted range of motion, and an X-ray showed a chip of bone torn off (avulsion fracture) and an effusion (fluid) in the joint. In order to rule out the possibility of a joint mouse (loose body) of cartilage in the elbow joint that would not be apparent on X-ray, an MRI was ordered. No such loose body was found, so Stanley was spared the necessity of an operation (surgical removal of a loose body, usually through an arthroscope).

Stanley was given a sling for a brief period of time, and his activity was restricted for several months, allowing the soft tissue injuries and avulsion chip to heal. During this time pain and inflammation were treated with a low-dose NSAID. At the end of this period, Stanley was pain-free, and rehabilitative exercises to strengthen the elbow were started. He missed the remainder of the baseball season but will be allowed to pitch again next year, although his time on the mound will be restricted. His team didn't take the state title (they came in third), but Stanley doesn't have to worry about a disabling chronic elbow condition and he may yet go on to pitch in the majors.

QUESTIONS AND ANSWERS—THE ELBOW

Q: Why does the elbow stiffen and lose function so easily after even a minor injury?

A: As we have seen, the elbow is actually three joints in one. Because the movements of these joints are interlinked, any change in the state of one of them can affect the others. This is why the elbow is prone to stiffness with even minor injury.

Q: Is a cast always necessary for the treatment of an elbow injury?

A: It depends on the injury. Generally, some sort of splint may be necessary for a brief period of time, but many elbow injuries can then be treated in a sling to encourage early motion and avoid stiffness.

Q: Are elbow injuries dangerous in children?

A: Very much so. Because there are many bone growth zones around the elbow, injury to any of these growth zones can cause arrest of growth or abnormal growth of the bones at the elbow, leading to deformity with significant functional loss. Because there are so many growth zones at the elbow, comparable X-ray views are taken of the injured and uninjured sides. By comparing X-rays of the injured elbow with those of the uninjured elbow, minimal displacement of bones can be detected.

Q: Is fusion of the elbow a disabling condition?

A: An elbow with normal movement is always better than one that has limited motion. However, a condition called congenital radial-ulnar fusion can be present from birth. People with this condition compensate for lack of forearm pronation and supination by moving their shoulder, and they seem to function very well. Complete loss of the flexion-extension ability of the elbow is a serious disability. Loss of flexion and extension from whatever cause at the extremes of movement, still maintaining a functional range of flexion-extension movement in between, is less of a problem.

The last stop in our "journey through the joints" is at the wrist and hand. So let's now see how these biomechanical marvels work.

12

The Wrist and Hand

"The hand that rocks the cradle
Is the hand that rules the world."
William Ross Wallace
The Hand That Rocks the Cradle
Stanza I

The eight bones of the wrist—the carpal bones—articulate with each other and with the far ends of the radius and ulna. They provide a variety of movement that, together with the other joints of the upper extremity, serve to position the hand in space so it is able to perform almost unbelievable feats of dexterity. It has been said that "... All human art is the increment of power of the hand" (John Fiske, *The Destiny of Man*, Ch. VII). The human hand is unique among animals in that the thumb can touch each finger. More of the brain is committed to movements of the hand than to any other motor task. The hand grips most efficiently with the wrist in extension (bent back). The fingers flex when the wrist is in this position, and they flex some 25,000,000 times during your lifetime to hold and manipulate a prodigious variety of objects. Conversely, the fingers will naturally extend with the wrist in flexion (bent forward).

GRASP AND GRIP

In contrast to the other digits, the index finger is able to function independently. Generally speaking, the side of the hand toward the radius is responsible for skilled precision movements such as pinch grip (thumb and index finger) and three-finger chuck grip (thumb, index, and middle fingers). The ulnar side of the hand is responsible for power grip. A pencil grasped between the index finger and the thumb can easily be removed. However, it is more difficult to retrieve when held between the ring finger and the little finger and the palm. The adroit movement of turning a key in a lock is much easier using the thumb and index finger than with any other combination of fingers or a finger and the thumb.

ANATOMY

There are arches in the hand similar to those in the feet. A *transverse* arch lies at the level of the wrist, and a *longitudinal* arch lies along the palm. The thumb is responsible for approximately 50 percent of hand function, and loss of a thumb in an industrial accident is granted at least a 50 percent disability. Set at a 90° angle to the rest of the fingers, the *metacarpal* of the thumb articulates in a saddle joint that enables significant motion and function. The muscles of the thumb at the *thenar* (thumb) eminence provide the thumb with a strong grip and grasp. The tendons, nerves, and other soft tissue structures for the palm enter the hand through the *carpal tunnel*, which is formed by a ligament—the transverse volar ligament—that spans the carpal bones at the wrist.

There are 27 bones in the hand and wrist. Those of the hand proper are labeled with the oxymoron "short long bones." The eight wrist bones, or carpals, articulate so as to provide smooth motion at the wrist, between the long bones of the forearm (the radius and the ulna) and the metacarpal bones of the palm, one for each finger. The thumb has two additional bones, called phalanges, and the other four fingers each have three. The term *phalanges* comes from the Greek for a band of soldiers drawn up for battle (Figure 12-1).

The equilateral spiral, a logarithmic curve, perfectly illustrated in the shell of the chambered nautilus and the shape of the egg, allows for the almost limitless ability of the hand to grasp. This curve is determined by intra-articular ratios of the small bones of the hand, which closely follow a *Fibonacci sequence* (0, 1, 1, 2, 3, 5, 8, 13 ...), in which each number is the sum of the two digits that precede it. The ratio (1:1.618) that

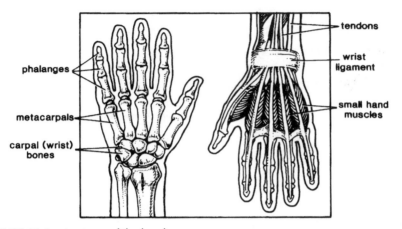

FIGURE 12-1   Anatomy of the hand.

this curve expresses is also seen in the golden rectangle of classical Greek architecture. Nature has accordingly fitted man with a superb instrument to serve an exquisite diversity of function and expression.

Mobility of the joints of the hand and wrist is ensured by a variety of ligaments and other fibrous structures that align and stabilize the bones. Ligaments alone normally are not responsible for holding joint surfaces together. This is because a ligament is a set of collagen fibers, which, like a string, can exert a reactive force only if stretched. However, an individual ligament can stop a movement that tightens it. When at rest, the bones of a joint are held together by the action of muscles and gravity. The small intrinsic muscles of the hand provide keenly tuned motor function, permitting very fine movement with great strength. The hand is also provided with an unusual array of sensory nerve endings that detect pressure, temperature, pain, and position (Fig 12-2).

FUNCTION

The human hand is unique in that the thumb can be brought to each finger. This *opposition* has played an integral part in human development. It is our ability to oppose our thumbs that grants us the skill to grasp tools and perform other functional tasks with our hands, distinguishing us from our primate

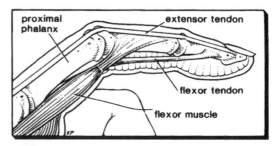

FIGURE 12-2   Normal finger anatomy.

cousins, the large apes. Proper function of the hand requires the ability to grasp and release the grip. Function is broadly categorized into power grasp (prehension), large cylindrical and small cylindrical holding, hooking, fine fingertip opposition, and bringing all the fingertips together in the form of a chuck. These skills enable the human hand to perform its many tasks.

What is most remarkable is that the hand possesses two distinct grips. For example, two balls can be separately held by different parts of a single hand. A bottle can be held and its cap unscrewed by the same hand. This dexterity adds dimensions to the operations of the human hand far beyond those of simpler functions. Even the appellation "surgeon" is derived from the Greek "cheir" (hand) plus "ergon" (work).

In carrying out its many duties, the hand is prone to accident and injury. The soft tissues can be bruised or cut. Falls can produce sprains, strains, and fractures of the wrist or fingers. The hand also can be the site of any kind of trauma or disease, including all varieties of arthritis.

Bony injuries to the wrist and hand, and soft tissue injuries of the hand, such as fingertip crush, fingertip loss, and lacerations, are covered in some detail in my other book *All About Bone* (Demos, 1998). Here we consider those medical conditions involving either directly or obliquely the joints of the wrist and hand.

FRACTURES

A *Colles fracture* is a break at the end of the two forearm bones (radius and ulna) that may extend into the wrist. This fracture often occurs with a fall on an outstretched hand. The wrist is

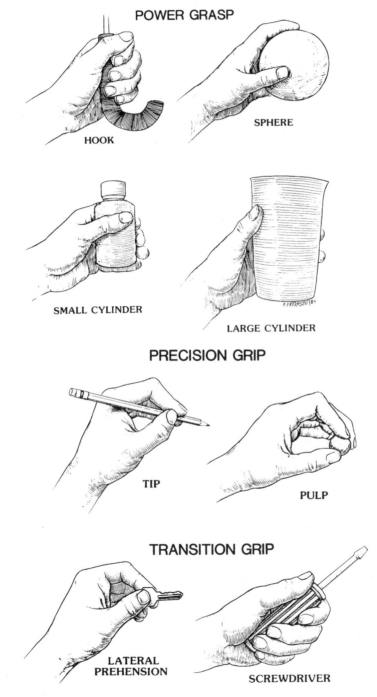

POWER GRASP

HOOK

SPHERE

SMALL CYLINDER

LARGE CYLINDER

PRECISION GRIP

TIP

PULP

TRANSITION GRIP

LATERAL
PREHENSION

SCREWDRIVER

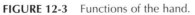

FIGURE 12-3   Functions of the hand.

deformed and has the shape of a dinner fork. If the fracture is in good position, treatment is simple and only a cast is required. If displaced or comminuted (many pieces), a closed or open reduction with metallic fixation may be required.

Fractures of the phalanges or metacarpals can also involve their joints and are similarly treated. When the fingers are jammed against a solid object, bony projections at the end of the phalanges, called condyles, may break or chip. Reduction, either closed or open, is necessary, followed by brief immobilization and early range of motion exercises to regain mobility. It is important to correct rotational displacement when setting fractures of the fingers. Otherwise, they will fail to work synchronously when performing fine motor tasks.

Some fractures that require special attention are:

1. *Bennett's fracture*, a fracture of the base of the first metacarpal into the carpometacarpal joint, which usually requires an open reduction with pin fixation and ligamentous repair.

2. *Fractured scaphoid*—the scaphoid (navicular), so called because it has the appearance of a boat; Greek = scaphos or Latin = navicular (hence the word Navy) is the carpal bone most frequently fractured. A fractured scaphoid can be serious because it involves joints in the wrist and because the carpal scaphoid has a minimal blood supply that, if interrupted, can lead to necrosis (death) of a portion of the bone. It can be difficult to diagnose with certainty. Every bad wrist sprain should be treated as a fracture of the scaphoid and immobilized in a cast until proven otherwise. A fractured scaphoid often requires open reduction and compression screw fixation. Sometimes this is augmented with a bone graft. Even when diagnosed early and treated correctly, a scaphoid fracture may fail to unite, causing chronic pain and considerable wrist disability.

3. *Intra-articular fracture* at the distal (far end) radius into the wrist requires accurate reduction and fixation with early mobilization to avoid the almost certain occurrence of traumatic arthritis at this joint.

4. A boxer's fracture is a break at the neck of the metacarpal with angulation of the metacarpal head

into the palm. It frequently is seen when someone strikes a hard surface with a clenched fist, breaking the bone at the knuckle. Almost all boxer's fractures are treated by closed reduction and casting for three to six weeks.

With any fracture of the hand or wrist, the arm should be elevated to decrease swelling after reduction. The fingers must be moved to maintain circulation and motion. The shoulder should also be exercised so it does not become stiff. Any unusual finger swelling, pain, discoloration (paleness or blueness), paralysis, or tingling (these are the five P's—puffiness, pain, pallor, paralysis, and paresthesia [pins and needles feeling]) should be reported immediately because they are indications that the cast is too tight and may require splitting for relief.

Dislocations of the finger joints, including the thumb, are frequently seen in an emergency room. Closed reduction usually is feasible unless soft tissue is interposed, in which case surgery may be necessary.

A patient may have persistent pain at the distal radioulnar joint because of a malunion of a wrist fracture or rheumatoid arthritis. The treatment is surgical, with excision of the distal ulna or reconstruction of the joint.

Infections of the joints of the wrist or hand are medical or surgical emergencies that must be treated with all dispatch. Appropriate antibiotics, rest, and heat, as well as early surgical drainage of an abscess before serious damage has occurred, are necessary.

SPRAINS

Sprains of the joints of the wrist and hand are common. X-rays may reveal separation of one or several wrist bones. This must be corrected by manipulation or surgery. A plaster cast often will hold the corrected position until healing is complete, but an operation with pin fixation sometimes is required.

A sprain can occur in any finger joint. A common injury is a tear of one of the *collateral* (side) ligaments of the thumb. These ligaments run along the base of the thumb, stabilizing it as it moves. Again, such sprains often are successfully treated by immobilization in a splint or cast, but surgical repair may be performed if a ligament is severely torn.

"Gamekeeper's thumb" is an injury, often a tear, of the ulnar (inside) collateral ligament of the thumb. Gamekeepers used to kill animals such as rabbits by snapping their necks between their thumb and index finger, stretching and injuring this ligament in the act. Today it is an athletic injury that most often occurs in skiing, from improper use of the ski pole, or in football, from blocking with the hands or falling on the thumb. An operation to repair the torn ligament is the treatment of choice.

An avulsion of the extensor tendon with or without a small chip of bone causing the fingertip to drop is called *mallet finger*. This frequently happens when one attempts to pull sheets tight while making a bed. Doing this involves forceful bending of the fingertips, and when the finger is suddenly released, the injury at the distal (far) interphalangeal joint can occur. Treatment is by splinting the fingertip straight for at least six weeks. Surgical correction occasionally is necessary.

GANGLION CYST

A *ganglion cyst* contains viscous fluid. It can occur anywhere in the hand or indeed about other joints, but it usually is found at the wrist. A ganglion cyst usually is in continuity with the joint or a tendon sheath. A tender lump appears that may alter in size. Diagnosis can be confirmed by decompressing the cyst through aspiration of the viscous, mucus-like fluid it contains. Injection of steroid medication into the cyst after aspiration sometimes prevents recurrence. Many ganglion cysts are self-limited, but definitive treatment often is available only through excision. This must be deep enough to remove the source of the ganglion cyst in the synovial sheath of the tendon or wrist joint itself. Otherwise the cyst will recur, as it does in 35 percent of operated cases.

RHEUMATOID ARTHRITIS

The hands are commonly involved in rheumatoid arthritis. Synovitis of the tendon sheaths and the joints occurs, particularly at the metacarpal phalangeal joints. The fingers drift toward the ulna. The involved joints may be destroyed and dislocate. Treatment is surgical, involving soft tissue excision and reconstruction as well as replacement of diseased joints by artificial ones of plastic or metal.

CARPAL TUNNEL SYNDROME

Although either the median nerve or the ulnar nerve entering the hand may be compressed, causing weakness and numbness, the most common nerve compression syndrome in the hand is *carpal tunnel syndrome*, which results from pressure on the median nerve as it enters the hand deep to the palmar surface of the wrist. To gain access to the fingers, the nerve must pass underneath a bridge of thick fibrous tissue called the *transverse volar carpal ligament*, which arches between several carpal bones to form the roof of a recess called the carpal tunnel. Tendons also pass through the tunnel, which makes the anatomy rather tight. Anything pressing into or causing swelling in this space can squeeze the nerve at the wrist.

Carpal tunnel syndrome is a frequent cause of work-related disability. However, recent studies report that the symptoms of carpal tunnel syndrome actually are quite common in the general population, particularly in women aged 65 to 75, in whom the prevalence is almost four times higher than in men.

The "repetitive strain syndrome" seen in typists or computer technicians is well known. Workers who use tools should try to keep their wrists in a neutral position, avoiding unusual strain by using a firm grip at all times. Frequent rest periods, minimizing repetitive tasks, support of the forearm while typing or using a computer, reducing force and speed in wrist movement, and conditioning exercises all help prevent carpal tunnel syndrome.

The syndrome is characterized by pain in the wrist with numbness of the thumb, index, and middle fingers. Symptoms often are worse at night. Other than repetitive strain, causes include the wear and tear of aging, bone dislocation and fracture causing bone to protrude into the carpal tunnel, arthritis, or fluid retention, which produces swelling in the tissues of the carpal tunnel, including the nerve itself. This occurs most often during pregnancy, with symptoms subsiding after delivery.

Examination for carpal tunnel syndrome includes physical tests such as gently tapping over the nerve, which induces a mild electrical shock–like feeling in the involved fingers (Tinel's sign), and positioning the wrist in a flexed (bent down) position, which quickly aggravates the numbness of the fingers (Phalen's sign). X-rays rule out contributing bony conditions. Electrical tests include a nerve conduction velocity test that measures the speed of electrical conduction along the nerve (it is reduced in carpal tunnel syndrome) and an electromyogram revealing abnormalities in the muscles at the base of the thumb. *Thermography*, the measurement of heat radiating from the hand, also is useful in the diagnosis of the condition.

The treatment of carpal tunnel syndrome includes resting the hand with a splint, antiinflammatory medication, occasionally diuretics or vitamin B_6, and often the injection of a steroid drug directly into the carpal tunnel in an attempt to decrease swelling and inflammation in the tunnel itself.

Many cases of carpal tunnel syndrome respond to these conservative measures. Those that do not require a carpal tunnel release. This is a relatively simple operation, usually performed under local anesthesia, either directly visualizing the compressed nerve or operating through an endoscope. The median nerve is identified and protected as the transverse volar carpal ligament is transected, easing pressure on the nerve.

Postoperative recovery requires using a splint for approximately one week, elevation of the arm to prevent swelling, and rehabilitation exercises to improve strength in the hand.

ATHLETIC INJURY

Any repetitive athletic activity of the hand and wrist can cause pain and disability. For example, wrist pain is common in gymnasts (particularly in females because of relative ligamentous laxity), and elite rowers. In skeletally immature gymnasts, a widening of the distal radial growth plate may be seen, and in skeletally mature gymnasts, a short radius relative to the ulna is present. Such athletes should avoid bending and bearing weight on the upper extremities until the wrist is no longer painful on movement. Rowers should restrict their activity for two to three weeks, ice the affected area, and take an NSAID.

REFLEX SYMPATHETIC DYSTROPHY

Reflex sympathetic dystrophy is characterized by severe pain in the hand with swelling, stiffness and discoloration. These symptoms and findings are progressive. It usually is preceded by trauma at a joint just proximal to that in which the condition occurs. It can also occur in the foot.

Reflex sympathetic dystrophy is considered to be caused by abnormal sympathetic nerve reflex activity. It must be treated early and strenuously because it can easily become chronic, disabling, and resistant to all treatment. Vigorous exercises are initiated to restore strength and range of motion. Medications and injections (stellate ganglion block at the level of the C6–7 vertebrae) are used to interrupt the abnormal sympathetic reflex.

CASE REPORT—The Hand

Sylvia P., a 25-year-old secretary, had never experienced difficulty with her hands or wrists. Then she changed jobs. Her new position required her to work at a computer for eight hours a day, and although she was paid more and her benefits were greater, after six months she began to experience numbness in her thumb, index finger, and middle finger (worse in her dominant right hand), as well as some pain radiating up her forearm and a gradual weakness of grip. Sylvia ignored her symptoms for a while, assuming that they were merely due to a change in work habits. Besides, she was a little better over her weekend time off and her vacation. She finally became concerned and went to her doctor for help when she not only did not improve with time but also began to get worse and her pain and numbness awakened her at night.

On examination, the doctor found that gently tapping over the palmar side of her wrist caused a mild electrical shock–like feeling in the involved fingers (Tinel's sign), and positioning of the wrist in a flexed (bent down) position aggravated her symptoms (Phalen's sign). X-rays of Sylvia's wrists ruled out bony conditions that might be causing pressure on the (median) nerve. A nerve conduction velocity test, which measures the speed of electrical conduction along the nerve, showed reduced velocity across the wrist. An electromyogram, which reveals electrical abnormalities in muscles, was positive in the muscles at the base of the

continued on next page

---

thumb. The doctor diagnosed carpal tunnel syndrome, which is a "repetitive strain syndrome," a work-related disability because of abnormal prolonged positioning of the hands and wrists subjecting the median nerve to repeated strain and chronic pressure as it passes through the carpal tunnel to serve the hand.

Treatment of carpal tunnel syndrome includes putting the hand at rest, and Sylvia was given splints for her wrists. An NSAID was prescribed, and she was advised to take a medical leave from work for two weeks. Her condition improved somewhat with these measures, but because of residual annoying numbness and some pain on the right side, her right carpal tunnel was injected with a steroid drug in an attempt to decrease swelling and inflammation in the tunnel itself. She also was given a brief course of oral steroid medication that was reduced over a period of one week, after which acupuncture treatment was started. Sylvia's symptoms all but disappeared and she returned to work. Her employer modified her workstation by providing a chair and desk of appropriate height, which will keep her wrist positioned at neutral, as well as a forearm support to reduce wrist strain. Sylvia was permitted frequent brief rest periods. She also was shown how to minimize her repetitive tasks and decrease the force and speed of her wrist movement. Finally, she was given conditioning exercises for her wrist and hand.

Like many cases of carpal tunnel syndrome, Sylvia's responded to these conservative measures. If she had not improved under this program, she would have required a surgical release of her carpal tunnel, transecting the volar transverse carpal ligament to ease pressure on the median nerve.

QUESTIONS AND ANSWERS—THE WRIST AND HAND

Q: What are the important things to remember when giving first aid for a wrist or hand injury?

A: Some important things to remember are:

❑ If there is a wound and it appears at all serious, do not attempt to cleanse it; just apply pressure over a clean pad to control bleeding.

❑ The wrist can be splinted with any convenient material, such as a folded newspaper or a firm pillow. The hand can be splinted by placing a roll of bandage or other material into the palm and curving the victim's fingers around it. For severe injury to many fingers, you can separate the fingers by gauze or cloth dressing material and cover the entire hand with a clean towel or cloth or with an unused plastic bag.

❏ During transportation, the hand should be kept elevated above the level of the heart in order to reduce swelling. Only after an insect sting or a snakebite should the hand be kept hanging down after injury to decrease the circulation of venom.

❏ If a finger has been cut off and is salvageable, wrap it in gauze soaked in salt water and transport it on ice to the emergency room.

Q: Are there orthopaedic techniques to restore function to severely congenitally deformed hands or those that have been badly injured?

A: Yes. There are operations to fuse unstable joints, release contractures, transfer tendons to provide increased range of motion, and graft skin to cover wounds. When amputation is necessary, prostheses are available that not only are cosmetically acceptable but also can be motivated electrically or through muscle connections higher up in the arm.

Q: What is de Quervain's disease? Dupuytren's contracture?

A: Fritz de Quervain was a Swiss physician who first described tendinitis of the wrist affecting the tendons that connect the thumb to the muscles of the forearm, hence the eponym. Dupuytren's contracture was named after a famous nineteenth century French surgeon, Guillaime Dupuytren. The contracture consists of chronic scarring of the fascia of the palm, leading to painless bending of the fingers into the palm with locking of the finger joints. Its cause is uncertain and it chiefly affects adult men, often those of Irish or Scottish ancestry. Ex-President Ronald Reagan, a descendent of Irish immigrants, suffered from Dupuytren's contracture, and his hand was operated on to relieve this condition during his last few weeks in office.

Q: What situations can result in serious hand injuries?

A: The gravest hand injuries undoubtedly occur in industrial or agricultural accidents. Hands mangled in corn pickers or crushed in punch presses present challenging reconstructive problems to specialists in hand surgery.

Q: What is club hand?

A: Club hand occurs at the wrist and is analogous to club-foot. There are two types. *Radial* club hand involves an absence or hypoplasia (lack of growth) of the radius and associated musculature, which produces a lateral (to the outside) deviation of the hand. *Ulnar* club hand is caused by an absence or hypoplasia of the ulna. The radius often is shortened and bowed, finger deformities are common, and the hand is shifted toward the midline.

Club hand may be isolated or may be part of a generalized skeletal *dysplasia* (malformation). Management depends on the severity of the deformity and the presence of associated defects. Operations are available for soft tissue release, which will reposition and stabilize the hand and wrist over the end of the remaining forearm bone.

Q: What is the role of hand therapy in the treatment of hand and wrist injury?

A: Hand and wrist therapy is labor-intensive. Rehabilitation requires intense and prolonged effort by both the patient and a skilled hand therapist. The therapist provides custom splinting, specific exercises, and other measures to strengthen and mobilize the injured member. The specialized knowledge of the hand therapist of wound healing, the influence of scars on movement, controlled tissue stress, and the like, are essential in the postsurgical management of the patient with a hand or wrist injury.

Q: What is Kienböck's disease?

A: Dr. Robert Kienböck, an Austrian radiologist, first described avascular necrosis (interrupted circulation leading to bone death) of the carpal lunate bone in 1910. The exact cause is not known, but anatomic variation of the bone, insufficient blood supply, and chronic repeated trauma may contribute to its onset. It occurs in young and middle-aged adults. Symptoms include wrist pain and stiffness; swelling and weakness may occur. X-rays show degeneration and increased density of the bone. Treatment depends on the stage of the disease. Early cases can be managed by lengthy cast immobilization.

Various operations to reduce stress on the lunate or to neovascularize the dead bone are available. When collapse of the bone is complete, treatment is directed toward creating carpal stability through a fusion operation at the wrist.

13

What About the Future?

The new decade promises momentous advances in the treatment of musculoskeletal disorders, thanks to the commencement of the Bone and Joint Decade (2000–2001). The Bone and Joint Decade is a global campaign to advance the understanding and treatment of orthopaedic disorders through education and research. Its worldwide goals include increasing funding for research and seeking cost-effective methods of prevention and treatment of bone and joint disease.

The cutting edge of basic science and clinical research has already discovered new techniques for the management of joint disease. Some examples include:

❑ Arthroscopic techniques are being used for surgery to almost any joint. There is even a way to perform an ankle fusion through the arthroscope.

❑ A microdecompressing (microscopic operation) procedure has been developed for spinal surgery. Spinal fusion can now be accomplished through small skin incisions, the so-called percutaneous route.

❑ Artificial intervertebral discs of stainless steel have been used to replace damaged discs in the cervical spine.

❑ Chronic low back pain accompanied by muscle spasm has been successfully treated with injections of attenuated botulinum toxin (Botox).

❑ Laser energy has been shown to induce collagen short-ening, tightening the capsular ligaments of a loose shoul-der, and thermal energy has been effective in shrinking the tissues in the lax shoulder or the loose ankle.

❑ Computerized operative planning and prosthetic design and sizing have been developed. With this technique, anatomic data are programmed and the surgery and implant are customized to fit each patient.

❑ The addition of some of the newer antibiotics to bone cement has decreased the risk of postoperative infection in joint replacement surgery.

❑ Bone morphogenic protein has been shown to expedite fusion of bone grafts in an animal model. Human studies are in the offing.

❑ In another animal experiment the biological activity of the intervertebral disc was modulated by transfer of a human growth factor through a virus. This transfer genetically modified the cells of the disc to produce the growth factor. Such molecular engineering holds the promise for the future treatment of human disease through molecular genetic technology.

❑ Laboratory studies of the formation of small bones and joints by tissue engineering has shown that well-defined whole-joint structures may be grown in the laboratory for transplantation.

❑ Another promising area of tissue engineering is the potential use of stem cells for the repair of damaged organs.

❑ Better understanding of the inflammatory response in rheumatoid arthritis has led to the development of bio-logical response modifiers that target for treatment key inflammatory and immunologic factors in this disease.

❑ Long-term pain relief and increased function have been provided to younger patients with osteoarthritis of the ankle through the surgical method of joint distraction.

❑ A tumor of an arm or leg is not always a warrant for amputation. Sophisticated surgical techniques for "limb sparing" using combinations of customized prostheses and bone grafts can often remove the tumor, yet save the extremity.

❏ Computer-generated, virtual reality, three-dimensional imaging, and robotic-assisted surgery will enable the surgeon to better visualize pathology and operate through minimal incisions. This will make it possible to perform surgery by remote control.

These are but a few examples of ongoing research being conducted in the field of bone and joint disease. And all of these techniques are becoming more and more available to practitioners worldwide through computer search engines on the World Wide Web for obtaining medical information for education and guidance.

The future holds many exciting discoveries. I sincerely hope that *All About Joints* has given you the knowledge to understand and appreciate these discoveries when they come about, as they most certainly will.

14

Summary

Let's review some of the key points about your joints covered in this book:

1. Your joints are a marvel. They enable you to stand, walk, run, and perform all of the tasks necessary to earn your living, maintain your life, express your individuality, engage in sport, perform in the arts, and achieve in the sciences.
2. All of this is accomplished through the variety of joints in your body, each one fashioned to meet its particular functional requirements.
3. Many forms of arthritis can occur. The most common types are osteoarthritis and rheumatoid arthritis. A variety of medical and surgical treatments are available to help these conditions.
4. Of all the therapies available for the treatment of joint injury and disease, exercise is far and away the most important treatment.
5. The hip is the deepest joint in the body and is subject to injury and aging. Early diagnosis of a child's hip problem is essential before serious disease evolves. Older adults with osteoporosis often fracture their hips. The adult hip was one of the first joints to be replaced by a total joint prosthesis.

6. The knee is the largest joint in the body. It frequently is the site of athletic injury. Arthroscopic techniques are available for the diagnosis and treatment of many knee problems.

7. The ankle joint can be the site of running injury, and is one of the most frequently sprained joints in the body. Fractures of the ankle must be treated aggressively because a stable and mobile ankle is essential for standing, walking, and running.

8. Correct shoes are important for proper function of the feet. Soft tissue problems must be rectified and fractures treated adequately to provide strong, painless feet.

9. The neck is often the site of tension and muscle spasm. Conservative treatment that includes physical therapy, support, and appropriate exercises usually will help most mechanical neck problems.

10. Proper postural habits are important in protecting your spine. This includes the use of appropriate chairs and a firm mattress. The early detection of spinal curvature in children can initiate treatment to prevent its progression. Most back pain in adults is mechanical in nature and responds to conservative measures such as heat, rest, support, medication, and exercise.

11. The shoulder is the most mobile joint in the body, sacrificing stability for range of motion. For this reason, it is most frequently dislocated. Treatment is directed toward maintaining this mobility so that the arm can continue to be used for all its tasks of daily living.

12. The elbow is a complex joint that readily loses mobility after injury. Elbow fractures should be treated with early motion.

13. Sprains of the wrist are common, but a fracture of one of the carpal bones should be suspected when the wrist is injured. Injuries and diseases of the hand must be treated aggressively to provide continued sensibility and motion in this important member, particularly the thumb.

Well, there you have it. We've taken a long look at all your joints. Continue to treat them sensibly and follow the suggestions given in this book, and they will continue to serve you well as you journey through the rest of your life.

15

A 12-Question Quiz to
See If You Know All
About Joints

1. An example of a ball-and-socket joint is the:
   a. shoulder
   b. knee
   c. hip
   d. elbow
   e. wrist

2. The most common type of arthritis is:
   a. rheumatoid arthritis
   b. osteoarthritis (degenerative arthritis)
   c. gout
   d. infectious arthritis
   e. psoriatic arthritis

3. A complete exercise program includes:
   a. endurance (aerobic) exercises
   b. strengthening (resistance) exercises
   c. range of motion (stretching) exercises

4. Older people fracture their hips because:
   a. they fall frequently
   b. they have osteoporosis
   c. they don't get enough vitamin C or E
   d. they overexercise

5. The two ligaments in the knee most commonly injured are:
   a. medial collateral ligament
   b. lateral collateral ligament
   c. anterior cruciate ligament
   d posterior cruciate ligament

6. The acronym R-I-C-E applied to the treatment of ankle sprains stands for:
   a. rest
   b. ice
   c. compression
   d. elevation

7. Properly fitted shoes should:
   a. hold the toes snug
   b. hold the heels snug
   c. be broken in
   d. have soft uppers
   e. require shoe inserts

8. The following can cause neck pain:
   a. emotional tension
   b. heartburn
   c. arthritis
   d. whiplash injury
   e. constipation

9. Surgery is indicated for back pain when:
   a. there is a disc space infection
   b. you have severe pain after bending
   c. a cauda equina syndrome has been diagnosed
   d. you have spinal stenosis
   e. you have a herniated disc with sciatica which has not responded to an adequate period of conservative treatment

10. The shoulder is actually a complex of:
    a. two joints
    b. three joints
    c. four joints
    d. five joints

11. Which nerve is usually at risk in elbow injuries?
    a. radial nerve
    b. ulnar nerve
    c. median nerve
    d. sciatic nerve

12. Which of the following statements regarding carpal tunnel syndrome is TRUE?
    a. It is a repetitive strain injury.
    b. All cases require surgery.
    c. It is caused by pressure on the median nerve.
    d. It causes numbness in the little finger.
    e. It can be diagnosed by electrical testing.

12. a, c, e
11. b
10. c
9. a, c, e
8. a, c, d
7. b, d
6. a, b, c, d
5. a, c
4. a, b
3. a, b, c
2. b
1. a, c

ANSWERS

Glossary

A

ABDUCTION: Movement of a part away from the body's midline or center, or the midline of an extremity.

ACHILLES TENDON: The largest tendon in the body. It connects the calf muscles to the heel bone.

ACROMION: A bony shelf from the shoulder blade that roofs the shoulder joint. The acromioclavicular (AC) joint connects the acromion to the clavicle.

ADDUCTION: Movement of a body part toward the body's midline or center, or the midline of an extremity.

AEROBIC EXERCISE: Exercise designed to increase oxygen consumption by the body.

AMPHIARTHROSIS: A type of joint, usually connected by cartilage, that permits only slight motion

ANALGESIC: A pain-relieving drug.

ANEURYSM: A sac formed by the thinning and dilatation of the wall of an artery, vein, or the heart. It is filled with blood or clotted blood, often forming a pulsating swelling.

ANODYNE: Pain relieving medication.

ANTERIOR CRUCIATE LIGAMENT: The crossed ligament inside the knee that lies toward the front (anterior) of the joint. Together with the posterior (rear) cruciate ligament, it helps stabilize the knee.

ANTERIOR DRAWER TEST: A test for detecting damage to the anterior cruciate ligament.

ARTHRITIS: Inflammation of a joint. This may be due to trauma, infection, degenerative processes, etc.

ARTHROGRAPHY (Arthrogram): An X-ray technique utilizing the injection of an absorbable contrast dye or air into a joint, allowing its contents to be visualized.

ARTHROPLASTY: Reconstruction of a joint

ARTHROSCOPY: A surgical technique to visualize and operate within a joint (often a knee) that utilizes a fiber-optic light source and a thin tube containing a miniature video system.

ATROPHY: Wasting of muscle or other body tissue.

AUTOSOMAL DOMINANT (TRAIT): Genetic trait expressed by one parent. Fifty percent of offspring are at risk for inheritance regardless of gender.

B

BAKER'S CYST: A large sac at the back of the knee, filled with fluid.

BIPEDALISM: Walking on two legs.

BONY ARCHITECTURE: The microscopic structure of bone that enables it to support body weight.

BONE FORMATION: The secretion and formation of bone matrix by osteoblasts that draws minerals from the blood stream to produce new bone.

BONE MASS: The amount of bone that comprises the skeleton. Bone mass is influenced by nutrition, exercise, and heredity. It reaches its peak at about age 35.

BONE MATRIX: The protein part of bone that gives bone its elastic feature. Bone matrix makes up about half of bone volume but only one-third its weight.

BONE MINERAL: The crystalline part of bone that lends bone its rigid character. Calcium and phosphorus are the principal minerals involved.

BONE REMODELING: A microscopic process of bone repair in which specialized cells (osteoblasts and osteoclasts) remove old bone, replacing it with new bone.

BONE RESORPTION: The process of bony remodeling in which osteoclasts remove old bone, allowing bone formation to then proceed.

BONE SCAN: Procedure used to determine bone mass and mineral density. It is also used to localize and measure uptake and intensity of certain radioactive markers in bone.

BRUISE: Skin discoloration (ecchymosis) produced by ruptured blood vessels beneath the skin, usually caused by a blow. Sometimes called a contusion.

BUNION: Swelling and/or deformity of the joint at the base of the great toe.

BUNIONETTE: Irritation of the base of the 5th metatarsal bone along the outside border of the foot, accompanied by pain, swelling, and redness.

BURSA: A moist sac located where body parts (tendon, muscle, bone, etc.) move against each other. Its purpose is to reduce friction. Bursitis is inflammation of a bursa.

C

CALCANEUS: Heel bone. Also called the os calcis.

CALCIUM SUPPLEMENT: Chemical calcium taken as a medicine (as distinguished from calcium in the diet).

CALLUS: Thickening of the skin over body parts that are subject to friction or pressure.

CANCELLOUS BONE: Spongy bone found in the shafts of the long bones, pelvis, and vertebrae. Contains the bone marrow. See Trabecular bone.

CARPAL TUNNEL: A tunnel deep to the palm side of the wrist containing tendons that connect the muscles of the forearm to the fingers. The median nerve passes through the carpal tunnel.

CARPALS: The eight small bones of the wrist.

CARTILAGE: The dense elastic connective tissue that covers the ends of bones at joints. Special cartilage also supports the nose and ears.

CHONDROMALACIA: Degenerative softening of the cartilage in a joint. Chondromalacia patella is due to wear and tear of the kneecap caused by malalignment injury or overuse.

CHYMOPAPAIN: The active principle of papaya fruit, used in chemonucleolysis, a surgical technique in which chymopapain is injected to dissolve the center of a ruptured disc.

CLAVICLE: Collarbone.

CLUBFOOT: Congenital deformity of the foot and ankle, in which the foot is bent down and in (talipes equinovarus).

COCCYX: Tailbone.

COLLAGEN: The principal protein of bone, as well as tendons, skin, ligaments, and cartilage.

COLLATERAL LIGAMENTS: Ligaments that run along the side of the joint. In the knee the lateral (outside) collateral ligament and the medial (inside) collateral ligament connect the femur to the tibia and provide stability by preventing the knee from moving sideways.

COMMINUTED (FRACTURE): Broken or crushed into small pieces.

COMORBIDITY: Additional (other) disease(s).

CONARTICULAR (SURFACES): Mating pairs of joint surfaces.

CONDYLE: An elliptical eminence at the end of a major bone.

CONNECTIVE TISSUE: The supporting framework of the human body. Skin, tendons, ligaments, fascia, bone, and cartilage are all connective tissues. Collagen is the principal protein of connective tissue.

CONTRAST BATHS: Alternating cold and warm baths used to reduce swelling and pain.

CORN: A callus occurring between or on top of the toes. Between the toes it is often called a soft corn.

CORTICAL BONE: Dense bone that makes up the outer walls of a bone. The shafts of long bones (radius and ulna, humerus, tibia and fibula, femur) are comprised of cortical bone.

CREPITUS: The crackling sound produced by the rubbing together of the dry synovial surfaces of joints, or the fragments of a fractured bone.

CT: Computerized (axial) tomography—A specialized x-ray technique that visualizes sections of the body.

CYST: A fluid-filled sac.

D

DEBRIDEMENT: Removal of degenerated debris from a joint, a wound, or elsewhere in the body.

DELTOID: The triangular muscle that covers the shoulder and upper arm. The deltoid raises the arm from the body.

DE QUERVAIN'S DISEASE: Tendinitis of the wrist that affects the tendons connecting the muscles of the forearm to the thumb.

DIARTHROSIS: Freely movable joint.

DIETARY CALCIUM: Calcium supplied by food.

DISC: The fibrous tissue spacer found between vertebrae.

DISCOGRAM: Imaging technique in which absorbable radiopaque dye is injected directly into the disc. In this way, diagnostic pain can be elicited and pathology visualized.

DISEASE: "Lack of ease"—A condition of pathology in the body.

DISLOCATION: The complete displacement of bones meeting at a joint. If the displacement is only partial, it is called subluxation.

DORSIFLEX: To flex the foot or hand backwards.

DUPUYTREN'S CONTRACTURE: Scarring of the palmar fascia that causes contracture, bringing the fingers into the palm.

E

EFFUSION: Swelling in a joint caused by an accumulation of fluid or blood.

EMG: Electromyography (electromyogram)—a technique for visualizing and measuring the electrical activity of muscle.

ENZYME: A specialized protein that acts as a catalyst in metabolic chemical reactions within living organisms.

EPIPHYSIS: A growth center occurring near the end of a bone.

ESTROGEN: The female sex hormone, produced principally by the ovaries.

EXTENSION: Straightening a joint.

F

FASCIA: The tough fibrous covering that encloses muscles. Inflammation of fascia is called fasciitis.

FEMUR: The thigh bone. This is the body's largest bone.

FIBROSITIS: A condition characterized by muscle pain and stiffness.

FIBULA: The thin outer bone of the leg.

FLEXION: Bending a joint.

FRACTURE: Breakage of a bone or cartilage.

G

GAMEKEEPER'S THUMB: Injury to the ligaments at the base of the thumb, where the web between the thumb and index finger begins.

GANGLION: A fluid-filled cyst that originates from a joint or a tendon sheath.

GASTROCNEMIUS: The muscle of the calf that, along with the soleus muscle, connects to the Achilles tendon.

GAUCHER'S DISEASE: A disease of lipid metabolism that affects the organs of the body as well as bone. Involvement of the hip joint can result in necrosis of the head of the femur.

GLYCOGEN: A large chemical molecule built of sugar. Glycogen is the body's major reserve of carbohydrate used for energy.

GLUCOSE: Chemical constituent of glycogen. A sugar whose utilization is controlled by insulin.

GOUT: A metabolic disease in which an excess of uric acid is produced, characterized by acute joint inflammation.

GREATER TROCHANTER: The knob of bone at the upper outer end of the femur.

H

HALLUX VALGUS: Bunion.

HALLUX RIGIDUS: Arthritis of the joint at the base of the great toe that results in stiffness and pain.

HAMSTRINGS: Muscles of the back of the thigh.

HEEL SPUR: A bony spike extending forward from the bottom of the heel bone.

HERNIATED DISC: Rupture of a disc between two vertebrae. This often causes compression of the spinal nerve roots with pain running down the leg (sciatica).

HIP POINTER: A bruise due to a blow on the bony ridge of the pelvis.

HORMONE: A chemical substance produced by an organ or gland that is carried by the blood to other organs, which are then metabolically stimulated by that substance.

HUMERAL EPICONDYLE: The lateral humeral epicondyle is the bony bump on the outside of the elbow. This is the location of the irritation that causes "tennis elbow." The medial humeral epicondyle lies on the inside of the elbow and is the location of discomfort in "little league elbow" or "golfer's elbow."

HUMERUS: The bone of the upper arm.

HYPER-: A prefix meaning excessive.

HYPO-: A prefix meaning less.

I

IDIOPATHIC: Without known cause.

IONIC: Relating to an ion, an atom, or a molecule carrying an electric charge.

ISOMETRIC EXERCISE: Exercise that does not involve any movement of a limb or joint.

-ITIS: A suffix meaning inflammation.

J

JOINT: The place where two bones are joined.

JOINT CAPSULE: The fibrous tissue that encloses a joint.

JOINT SPACE: The space enclosed within the joint. Joints can have a synovial lining, which produces synovial fluid.

L

LAMINECTOMY: Spinal surgery that involves the removal of bone from the back (lamina) of the spinal column, usually performed as part of the removal of a ruptured disc, spinal tumor, or other impingement on the spinal cord or its nerves.

LIGAMENT: A tough fibrous band that connects bone to bone.

LOADING: The pressure or burden placed on a joint during weight bearing or exercise. Also, *unloading* (reducing the pressure) and *hyperloading* (increasing the pressure).

LORDOSIS: The normal front to rear curve of the low back. Sway-back is hyperlordosis.

LUPUS (ERYTHEMATOSUS): (Latin = wolf) A group of connective tissue disorders that primarily affect women aged 20 to 40 years. It is of unknown etiology but is thought to be an autoimmune condition. The disorder is marked by a wide variety of abnormalities, including arthritis, kidney disease, central nervous system manifestations, blood disorders, and skin lesions.

M

MALUNION: Literally, bad union, in which a fracture is not properly set and unites with the fracture fragments angulated, rotated, severely overlapped and shortened, or otherwise poorly aligned.

MECHANORECEPTOR: Receptors found in muscle, tendons, and soft tissues near joints that are excited by mechanical pressure or distortions such as muscular contraction. Mechanoreceptors send signals to the central nervous system, keeping the body informed of the position of the joints.

MENISCI: Thick cartilage half-rings that cushion the knee, providing shock absorption. The operation of partial or total removal of a meniscus is called a meniscectomy.

MENOPAUSE: Permanent cessation of ovarian function. This occurs naturally when the ovaries stop producing estrogen, usually in the early 50s.

MESODERM: (Gr. middle – skin) The middle layer of the three primary germ layers of the embryo. From it are derived the connective tissue, bone and cartilage, and muscle, as well as blood and blood vessels, lymphatics, central nervous system precursors, pleura, pericardium, peritoneum, kidneys, and gonads.

METACARPALS: The five hand bones that connect the wrist bones to the bones of the fingers.

METATARSALGIA: Pain, usually on weight-bearing, in the area of the metatarsal heads (short or transverse arch) of the foot. The metatarsal arch can be collapsed.

METATARSALS: The five foot bones that connect the toes with the top of the foot.

MORBIDITY: Relative incidence of disease.

MORTALITY: Death.

MYELOGRAM: X-ray taken of the spine after injecting an absorbable radiopaque dye into the spinal fluid. In this way, a herniated disc or other space-occupying lesion can be identified.

MYOSITIS OSSIFICANS: A condition in which bone is formed within muscle. This occurs as the result of muscular damage secondary to trauma and bleeding.

N

NAVICULAR: A boat-shaped bone found in both the wrist and the foot. In the wrist it is sometimes called the scaphoid.

NCV: Nerve Conduction Velocity—Diagnostic technique that measures the conduction of electricity along a nerve. Useful in diagnosing nerve pressure syndromes and other nerve pathology.

NEUROFIBROMATOSIS: A familial condition characterized by developmental changes in the nervous system, muscles, bones and skin. Soft tissue tumors are distributed over the entire body in association with areas of hyperpigmentation.

NONUNION: Failure of a bone to unite after fracture.

NSAID: <u>N</u>on-<u>S</u>teroidal <u>A</u>nti-<u>I</u>nflammatory <u>D</u>rug. A drug, not related to cortisone, that suppresses inflammation in the body and relieves pain.

O

OCCUPATIONAL THERAPY (OT): Therapy directed toward restoring function after disease or injury. Occupational therapy rehabilitates the patient to perform tasks of daily living.

OLECRANON: The end of the ulna that extends behind the elbow joint.

OLECRANON BURSITIS: Inflammation of the elbow bursa over the olecranon.

OPPOSITION: Thumb pinching.

ORTHOPAEDICS: That medical specialty that deals with the diagnosis and treatment of disorders of the musculoskeletal system. This includes bones, joints, ligaments, muscles, tendons, and other related structures.

ORTHOTICS (sing. orthosis): Appliances designed to balance the foot. Also used as a synonym for brace.

OSGOOD-SCHLATTER'S DISEASE: Tendinitis at the end of the patellar tendon. It appears to be associated with growth plate immaturity at the front of the tibia. It usually affects vigorous boys between the ages of 10 and 16. It is self-limited.

OSTEOARTHRITIS: The most common form of arthritis. It usually involves weight-bearing joints. It is characterized by cartilage destruction and bony overgrowth.

OSTEOBLAST: Bone-producing cell.

OSTEOCHONDRITIS DISSECANS: A condition that causes a fragment of bone and its overlying cartilage to degenerate. If the blood supply is entirely lost, it may loosen and separate into a joint, often the ankle or knee.

OSTEOCLAST: Cell that removes bone.

OSTEOCYTE: The basic cell within the structure of bone.

OSTEOGENESIS: Bone production.

OSTEOGENESIS IMPERFECTA: A disorder caused by the defective formation of collagen, resulting in shortened, deformed, brittle bones.

OSTEOMALACIA: A disease in which bone matrix fails to mineralize. Although produced by many factors, it can be caused by vitamin D deficiency in adults.

OSTEONECROSIS: Death of bone.

OSTEOPENIA: Reduced bone mass, for whatever reason.

OSTEOPOROSIS: Loss of mineral from bone resulting in bony weakening and a predilection for fracture.

OSTEOTOMY: A surgical procedure that involves breaking a bone and resetting it, often performed to more evenly distribute pressure across a joint.

P

PARATHYROID HORMONE: A hormone produced by the parathyroid glands, which lie next to the thyroid in the front of the neck, that is essential for calcium metabolism.

PATELLA: Kneecap.

PELVIS: The bony ringlike structure (also called the pelvic girdle) to which the legs and the spine are attached.

PERIOSTEUM: The dense fibrous tissue that covers the surface of bone and from which circumferential bone growth occurs.

PERTHES DISEASE (Legg-Calvé-Perthes disease): Necrosis of the bone of the head of the femur, usually found in young boys.

PES PLANUS: Flat feet.

PHALANGES: The bones of the toes and fingers.

PHYSICAL THERAPY: Rehabilitation that is directed to the prevention of disability and restoration of function following disease or injury. Physical therapy (PT) utilizes physical methods such as exercise, cold, and heat.

PHYSIS: (Gr. to generate) Growth plate found at the end of long bones.

PLANTAR FASCIA: The dense fibrous tissue running along the inside of the sole of the foot from the heel to the base of the toes which maintains the long arch. Inflammation of this structure is called plantar fasciitis.

PLICAE: Thin membranous walls within the knee. These are developmental left-overs. They usually disappear at the end of fetal growth but sometimes remain, causing irritation in the knee.

POLYMYALGIA RHEUMATICA: This condition mostly affects people over 50. It is characterized by shoulder and hip muscle pain and stiffness and a high sedimentation rate of the blood.

POPLITEAL: Refers to the back of the knee.

POSTERIOR: Toward the back of the body.

PROGNOSIS: Prediction of the outcome or recovery of a disease.

PROLOTHERAPY: Injection of a sclerosing solution into ligaments (usually of the back). This scars and tightens the soft tissue, providing stability to the bony elements.

PRONATION: Turning the hands with the palm downward. Pronation also refers to excessive inward rolling of the ankles.

PROPRIOCEPTION: Awareness of position.

PROSTAGLANDINS: Chemicals responsible for pain and swelling.

PSEUDARTHROSIS: False joint. When a fracture fails to unite, it can proceed to form a pseudarthrosis.

Q

QUADRICEPS: The large muscle group in the front of the thigh.

R

RADIUS: The outer bone of the forearm.

REDUCTION: The restoration of a displaced part of the body to its normal position. The 'setting' of a fracture involves reduction of the bony fragments to their anatomical pre-fracture position.

RHEUMATOID ARTHRITIS: The second most common form of arthritis. Rheumatoid arthritis is an inflammatory condition of the synovial lining of joints.

RHEUMATOLOGIST: A medical physician who specializes in the diagnosis and treatment of rheumatic diseases.

RICKETS: A childhood disease characterized by defective bone formation with severe deformities of the skeleton. Rickets is often due to a deficiency of vitamin D.

S

SACRUM (SACRED BONE): The triangular bone just below the lumbar vertebrae, formed usually by five fused vertebrae. The coccyx is attached distally to the sacrum.

SARCOPENIA: Lack of or wasting of muscle tissue.

SCAPULA: Shoulder blade.

SCIATICA: Irritation of the sciatic nerve, which is the large nerve that supplies much of the leg from the hip down.

SCOLIOSIS: A side to side curve of the spine.

SEDIMENTATION RATE: A laboratory blood test used to indicate inflammation in the body.

SESAMOID BONES: Tiny bones within tendons that lie under the great toe. Irritation of the sesamoid bones is called sesamoiditis. Strictly speaking, because it too lies within a tendon, the patella is a sesamoid bone.

SICKLE-CELL DISEASE: A disease caused by abnormal hemoglobin in the blood in which bony involvement may occur.

SNAPPING HIP: Popping at the outside of the hip joint. This is usually caused by a tendon snapping over bone.

SODIUM FLUORIDE: A chemical prescribed to strengthen bone.

SOMATICIZE: The tendency to express negative feelings and emotions through tension of musculoskeletal structures. This usually occurs in the neck, spine, and shoulders.

SPINAL COLUMN: The flexible bony column that extends from the skull through the low back. It surrounds and protects the spinal cord.

SPINAL FUSION: A surgical operation in which the spine is straightened and kept rigid, often through the use of metallic appliances augmented with bone grafts.

SPINAL STENOSIS: An arthritic condition, usually found in older individuals, in which the spinal canal is narrowed, causing pressure on the spinal nerves.

SPONDYLOLISTHESIS: The forward displacement of one vertebra over another, usually of the 4th lumbar over the 5th, or the 5th lumbar over the body of the sacrum. The condition is usually due to a developmental defect in the vertebral arch.

SPONDYLOLYSIS: A break in the continuity of the vertebral arch, leading to instability at that vertebral level.

SPRAIN: A stretch or tear of a ligament.

STERNUM: Breast bone.

STRAIN: A stretching injury to a tendon.

STRESS FRACTURE: A hairline fracture caused by stress to the bone. It is often too fine to appear on ordinary x-rays and requires a bone scan for diagnosis.

STRESS X-RAY: An x-ray taken while a joint is stressed.

SUPINATION: Applied to the hand, the act of turning the palm upward. Applied to the foot, raising the medial (inside) margin of the foot.

SYMPATHETIC (NERVOUS SYSTEM): That part of the autonomic nervous system that is not under voluntary control. The sympathetic nervous system supplies blood vessels, smooth muscles, and glands.

SYMPATHETIC DYSTROPHY OR REFLEX SYMPATHETIC DYSTROPHY (RSD): A painful condition characterized by swelling, discoloration, and osteoporosis of a hand or foot, often after a minor injury. Sympathetic dystrophies are due to dysfunction of the sympathetic nervous system. The wasting (atrophy) that occurs in sympathetic dystrophy is called Sudeck's atrophy.

SYNARTHROSIS: A fibrous joint, such as those found in the skull of an infant.

SYNDROME: A collection of signs and symptoms that characterize an abnormal condition.

SYNOVIAL FLUID: The thick colorless lubricating fluid contained within a joint or bursa.

SYNOVIAL MEMBRANE: The joint lining that produces synovial fluid. Inflammation of the synovium is called synovitis.

T

TALUS: The lowest ankle bone.

TENDON: Fibrous tissue cords attaching muscle to bone. Inflammation of a tendon is called tendinitis.

TENS: <u>T</u>ranscutaneous <u>E</u>lectrical <u>N</u>erve <u>S</u>timulation. A technique for pain relief by the stimulation of nerves through wires connected to the skin, powered by a small battery carried by the patient.

TERRIBLE TRIAD: A major knee injury that involves tearing of the medial meniscus and rupture of both the medial collateral and anterior cruciate ligaments.

THIXOTROPY: Property of changing the viscosity of a fluid with shaking or change of pressure.

TIBIA: The larger of the lower leg bones (the shin bone).

TOTAL JOINT REPLACEMENT: Surgery to replace a joint with metal and plastic components. Cemented and non-cemented types are available.

TRABECULAR BONE: The spongy bone that fills the ends of long bones, the central portion of the vertebrae, and the inside of flat bones.

TRACTION: Pull applied to a limb through the use of weights and pulleys.

U

ULNA: The inner bone of the forearm.

ULTRASOUND: High-frequency sound waves that are used for therapy. Ultrasound produces heat in deep body tissues. Ultrasound can also be used for diagnostic purposes (ultrasonography).

URIC ACID: A waste product of the body. An excess of uric acid can lead to gout.

V

VERTEBRAE: The small bones that make up the spinal column.

VITAMIN D: A substance that increases the capacity to absorb dietary calcium. It is not a true vitamin as it is produced in the human body when the skin is exposed to sunlight.

W

WEAVER'S BOTTOM: Ischial bursitis.

WHIPLASH: Flexion-extension injury of the neck, usually occurring to a passenger in a car involved in a rear-end collision

Suggestions for Further Reading

All About Bone, I.M. Siegel, Demos Medical Publishing, New York, 1998.

All About Muscle, I.M. Siegel, Demos Medical Publishing, New York, 2000.

The Ciba Collection of Medical Illustrations, Vol. 8. "Musculoskeletal System," Part I and Part II, Frank H. Netter, M.D., Ciba-Geigy Corporation, Summit, NJ, 1991.

Bones, Muscles and Joints, American Medical Association Home Medical Library, Medical Editor C.B. Clayman, The Reader's Digest Association, New York, Montreal, 1992.

The Random House Book of 1001 Questions and Answers about the Human Body, Trevor Day, Random House, New York, 1994.

Discovering the Human Body, Bernard Knight, Lippincott & Crowell, New York, 1980.

The Human Body ("The Skeleton"), K.E. Goldberg and editors of U.S. News Books, Washington, DC, 1982.

ADVANCED READINGS

Campbell's Operative Orthopaedics, 8th ed., edited by A.H. Crenshaw, M.D., Mosby Yearbook, St. Louis and Chicago, 1992.

Skeletal Trauma, 2nd ed., by Browner, Jupiter, Levine, and Prafton, W.B. Saunders, Philadelphia and London, 1998.

Surgery of the Musculoskeletal System, 2nd ed., edited by C. McCollister Evarts, Churchill-Livingstone, New York and London, 1990.

Copemann's Textbook of the Rheumatic Diseases, 6th ed., edited by J.T. Scott, Churchill-Livingstone, Edinburgh and London, 1986.

Diagnosis and Treatment of the Spine, P.T. Doswinkel, Aspen Publishers, Gaithersburg, MD, 1996.

The Textbook of Spinal Surgery, 2nd ed., edited by Editors- In-Chief K.H. Bridwell, R.L. DeWald, Lippincott-Raven, Philadelphia and New York, 1997.

The Shoulder, 2nd ed., edited by Rockwood and Matson, W.B. Saunders, Philadelphia and London, 1998.

Green's Operative Hand Surgery, 4th ed., edited by D.P. Green, R.N. Hotchkiss, W.C. Pederson, Churchill-Livingstone, New York and Edinburgh, 1999.

Surgery of the Knee, 2nd ed., edited by J.N. Insall, R. Windsor, W.N. Scott, M.A. Kelly, and P. Aglietti, Churchill-Livingstone, New York and Edinburgh, 1993.

Disorders of the Ankle, H. Kelikian, A. Kelikian, W.B. Saunders, Philadelphia and London, 1985.

Disorders of the Foot, edited by M.H. Jahss, W.B. Saunders, Philadelphia and London, 1982. The Child's Foot, M. Tachdjian, W.B. Saunders, Philadelphia and London, 1985.

The Adult Hip, edited by J. Callaghan, A.G. Rosenberg, H.E. Rubash, Lippincott-Raven, Philadelphia and New York, 1998.

The Shoulder and Neck, 2nd ed., J. Bateman, V. Fornisier, W.B. Saunders, Philadelphia and London, 1978.

The Elbow and Its Disorders, B.F. Morrey, W.B. Saunders, Philadelphia and London, 1985.

The Wrist and Its Disorders, 2nd ed., B. Lichtman, A. Alexander, W.B. Saunders, Philadelphia and London, 1997.

Practical Orthopedics, 4th ed., L.R. Mercier, Mosby–Yearbook, St. Louis and Baltimore, 1995.

Clinical Orthopedics, edited by E.V. Craig, Lippincott, Williams & Wilkins, Philadelphia and Baltimore, 1999.

The History of Orthopaedics, David LeVay, Parthenon Publishing, New Jersey, 1990.

Fundamentals of Pediatric Orthopaedics, L.T. Staheli, Raven Press, New York, 1992.

Chapman's Orthopaedic Surgery, 3rd ed., edited by M. W. Chapman, Lippincott Williams & Wilkins, Philadelphia and Baltimore, 2001.

Index

Note: Boldface numbers indicate illustrations.

Abduction, 4
Abnormalities in joints, 3
Absorbable (bioabsorbable, resorbable) fixation devices, 107–108
Acetabulum, 67, **69**
Achilles tendon, 119
Acromegaly, 14
Acromioclavicular joint, 165, 170–171
Active rest, 52
Acupuncture, 18, 157, 179
Adenosine triphosphate, 33
Adhesive capsulitis or frozen shoulder, 167–168, **171**
Aerobic exercise, 32–33, 51–52, 58
Aging and exercise, 32–34, 59, 61
Alexander method exercises, 56
Allograft, 20, 90, 96
Alternative treatments, arthritis, 18, 27
American Academy of Orthopaedic Surgeons, on back injury, 149

American Academy of Pediatrics, 61
American Physical Therapy Association, 41
Amphiarthroses, 4
Amputations, 204
Anemia, rheumatoid arthritis and, 22
Ankle, 20, 21, 105–110
    anatomy of 105, **106**
    arthritis in, 108, 109–110
    arthrodesis (fusion) surgery for, 108, 110
    calcaneus (heel bone) and, 105
    close-packed position, 6
    diabetes and, 110
    exercises for, 108
    fractures in, 106–108
    injuries to, 105–109
    ligaments of, 105
    osteochondritis dissecans in, 108
    questions and answers about, 109–110
    RICE therapy for injuries in, 106

running injury to, 108–109
sprains in, lateral ligament,
    106–107, 110
surgical treatment in, 107–108
talus bones of, 105
tibia and fibula in, 105
weight-bearing in, 105
Ankylosing spondylitis, 12
Ankylosis of joint, 29
Antibiotics, 204
Antinuclear testing, in arthritis,
    15
Antioxidants, 61
Arch of the foot, 112, 116–117,
    116
Arthritis, 9–30, 204
  acromegaly in, 14
  alternative treatments for, 18,
    20, 27
  in ankle, 108, 109–110
  ankylosing spondylitis and, 12
  ankylosis in, 29
  Bouchard's nodes in, 14
  cartilage degeneration in, 9–10,
    13, 14
  causes of, 13–14, 29
  childhood, 10
  corticosteriods for, 12, 16–17
  COX-2 inhibitors, 75
  creaking or grating noises in,
    15
  deformity in, 21
  degenerative (*See* osteo
    arthritis)
  diet and herbal remedies in, 19
  in elbow, 182–183
  exercise vs., 17–18, 29
  in foot, 122, 124
  forms of, 10
  giant cell arthritis and, 12
  gouty, **13**, 15, 24–26
  heat treatments in, 18
  Heberden's nodes in, 14
  hemorrhagic joint disease in, 28

in hip, 70, 75–83
infectious, 11, 28
inflammatory (*See* Rheumatoid
    arthritis)
inflammatory response and
    arthritis, 10–11, 204
in knee, 10, 88, 97–98, 102, 103
medication for, 14, 15–20, 22–23
muscle relaxants in, 17
in neck, 131, 134
nonsteroidal antiinflammatory
    drugs (NSAIDs), 75
osteo-, 12–20, **13**, 204
  acromegaly in, 14
  alternative treatments in, 18
  in ankle, 108
  Bouchard's nodes in, 14
  cartilage degeneration in, 13, 14
  causes of, 13–14
  corticosteriods for, 16–17
  creaking or grating noises in, 15
  diet and herbal remedies in, 19
  exercise vs., 17–18
  in foot, 124
  heat treatments in, 18
  Heberden's nodes in, 14
  in hip, 75
  magnet treatments for, 18–19
  medication for, 14, 15–20
  muscle relaxants in, 17
  in neck, 131, 134
  osteonecrosis and, 14
  prevalence of, 13–14
  process of, **13**
  sciatica in, 14
  in shoulder, 172–173, 174
  in spine, 151, 164
  stiffness in, 14–15
  stimulation of cartilage growth
    vs., 20–21
  surgery for, 19–20
  synovial fluid in, 15
  tests for, 15
  topical treatments for, 17

treatment of, 15–20
viscosupplementation in, 17
vitamin therapy for, 16
weight gain and, 17
weight-bearing joints in, 14
osteonecrosis and, 14
osteotomy and, 78
pain in, 10–12, 21, 22
pigmented villondular synovitis
   in, 29–30
polymyalgia rheumatica and, 12
prevalence of, 10, 13–14
process of, **13**
pseduogout and, 28–29
psoriatic, 28
psychogenic rheumatism and,
   12
questions and answers about,
   27–30
reactive, 27–28
rheumatic fever vs., 28
rheumatism and, 11
rheumatoid, **13**, 21–23, 204
autoimmune nature of, 22
in elbow, 182–183
in foot, 124
genetic therapy for, 23
hand deformities in, 21
in hip, 75
joint replacement surgery in, 23
joints involved in, 21
juvenile, 21
in neck, 131, 134
prevalence of, 22
in shoulder, 172–173
surgery for, 23
symptoms of, 21–22
synovectomy in, 23
synovial membrane degeneration in, 21
tests for, 22
toxin exposure and, 21
treatment of, 22–23
in wrist and hand, 194–195

sciatica in, 14
sedimentation rate test for, 12,
   22
in shoulder and, 172–173, 174
Sjögren's syndrome and, 28
soft tissue disorders in, 11–12
in spine, 146, 151, 164
stiffness in, 10, 12, 14–15, 21, 22
stimulation of cartilage growth
   vs., 20–21
surgical treatment of, 19–20,
   23, 29–30, 78
swelling in, 10, 21, 22
syndromes of, 27–28
synovial fluid in, 15
in temporomandibular joint, 29
treatment of, 15–20, 22–23
viscosupplementation in, 17
vitamin therapy for, 16
weight gain and, 17
weight-bearing joints in, 14
in wrist and hand, 193,
   194–195
Arthritis Foundation, 27
Arthrodesis (fusion) surgery, 78,
   108, 110, 148, 157, 174
Arthropathy, 28
Arthroscopic surgery, 89, 94, 96,
   97, 100, 203
Arthrosesis, knee, 99
Articular cartilage, 2–3, **2**, 9
Articular disc, 3
Articular processes of vertebrae,
   140–141
Articulation, 1, 2
Aseptic necrosis, hip, 85
Aspiration of joint fluid, 16–17,
   22, 74
Aspirin, 15, 16
Athletic fitness, 59–60
Autografts, 20
Autologous cartilage cell
   implantation, knee, 90
Avascular necrosis, hip, 71, 72

Avulsion fractures, elbow, 181
Azathrioprine, 22

Bacterial arthritis, 11
Baker's cyst, 94, 96–97
Balance exercises, 40–42, 65–66
Ball-and-socket joint (*See also*
    Hip; Shoulder), 4, **5**, 67, 165
Ballet and foot injuries, 11, 122,
    127
Bennett's fracture, 192
Blount's disease, 102
Body of vertebrae, 140, **142**
Bone, 9, 10
Bone and Joint Decade, 203
Bone cement, in replacement
    surgery, 84
Bone grafts and fusion (*See*
    Arthrodesis)
Bone morphogenic proteins, 148,
    204
Bone scans, 145, 154
Boosted lubrication, 10
Botulinum toxin (Botox) treat-
    ment, 124, 138, 203
Bouchard's nodes, 14
Bowleg (genu varum) condition,
    95, 102, 113
Bowler's thumb, 11
Boxer's fracture, 192–193
Braces, 102, 146
Brachial plexus, 173
Bunion joint, 24
Bunions (hallux valgus) and,
    121–123, 128
Burner or stinger shoulder injury,
    173–174
Bursae and bursitis, 11, 73–74,
    94, 121, 166–167, 177, 181

Calcaneal apophysitis (Sever's
    disease), 119

Calcaneus (heel bone), 105, 117
Calcium pyrophosphate dihy-
    drate, in arthritis, 29
Campbell, Wilis, 103
Capitulum, **178**
Capsaicin cream, 17
Capsule, 1, 2, **2**, 69, **178**
Capsulitis, 11
Carpal bones, 187, **189**
Carpal tunnel, 188, 195–196
Carpal tunnel syndrome, 195–196
Cartilage, 2–3, **2**, 11
    arthritis and, 9–20
    growth stimulation of, vs.
        arthritis, 20–21
    knee, 99
    osteoarthritis and, 13, 14
    spine and, 144
Cauda equina syndrome, 158
Celecoxib (Celebrex), 16
Cervical joint lock, 135–136
Cervical vertebrae, 140, **141**, 143
Cervicitis, 27
Charcot joint, 110
Chauffeur's knee, 95
Chemonucleolysis, 158
Childhood arthritis, 10
Chondrification, 3
Chondrocytes, 20
Chondroitin sulfate, 17
Chondromalacia patellae, 96
Chuck grip, 188
Circumduction, 4
Claudication, 12
Clavicle, 165, 170
Clinoril (*See* Sulindac)
Close-packed position of joint, 6
Club foot (congenital talipes
    equinovarus) in, 123–124
Club hand deformity, 200
Coccyx, 140
Colchicine, 26
Collagen, 9, 204
Collars, 132, 135

Collateral ligaments, knee, 88
Colles fracture, 190, 192
Compartment syndrome, 183
Components of a joint, **2**
Computed tomography (CT), 70, 94, 134, 138, 145, 154
Conarticular surfaces, 4
Congenital deformities, 3, 14
Congenital hip dislocation, 84
Congenital pseudarthrosis of clavicle in, 174
Congenital radial-ulnar fusion, 185
Congenital talipes equinovarus (clubfoot), 123–124
Conjunctivitis, 27
Connective tissue, 10
  Corns, 12
Corticosteroids, 12, 16–17, 22, 26, 71, 74, 157, 159
COX-2 inhibitors, 16, 75
Coxa plana (*See* Legg-Calvé-Perthes [LCP] disease)
Creaking or grating noises in joints, 15
Cross-training exercises, 54–55
Cruciate ligaments, knee, 88
Curvature (abnormal) of spine, 144–148, **147**
Cybex exercise machine, 100
Cycling as execs, 38
Cyclooxygenase-2, 16
Cyclophosphamide, 22
Cyclosporine, 22

Dancer's hip, 11
Dancing as exercise, 38–39
Daypro (*See* oxaprozin)
de Quervain's disease, 199
Debridement of arthritic joints, 19–20
Deformities of joints (*See also* Arthritis), 14, 21

Degenerative arthritis (*See* Osteoarthritis)
Development of joints, 3, 10
Developmental hip dysplasia (DDH), 71–72
Diabetes, 14, 110, 117–118
Diarthroses, 4
Diarthrosis joints, 68
Diathermy, 18, 132, 136
Diclofenate sodium (Voltaren), 16
Diet and exercise, 19, 61–62
Diflunisal (Dolobid), 16
Discectomy (removal of spinal disc), 151
Discitis, spine and, 145
Discs, vertebral discs, 142–143, **142**, 145
Dislocation (*See* Fractures and dislocations)
Disuse atrophy of muscles, 90
DNA testing, in arthritis, 15
Dolobid (*See* Diflunisal)
Dorsiflexion, 6
Down's syndrome, neck abnormalities, 132
Dupuytren's contracture, 199

Eastern (Asian)-style exercises, 55–56
Eddying of synovial fluid, 6
Effusions, 70
Elbow, 4, 14, 20, 177–185
  anatomy of, **178**
  arthritis in, 182–183
  avulsion fractures to, 181
  bones of, 177
  bursa and bursitis in, 177, 181
  capitulum in, **178**
  casts and splints for, 184
  in children, 184–185
  compartment syndrome in, 183
  congenital radial-ulnar fusion in, 185

exercises for, 179–180
extensor-supinator muscles of,
   177–178
flexor-pronator muscles of,
   177–178
fractures and dislocations in,
   181, 182
humeroradial joints in, 177
humeroulnar joint in, 177
humerus in, 177, **178**, 182
injuries to, 178–181,
   184–185
joint capsule of, **178**
joint replacement in, 183
lateral epicondylitis (tennis
   elbow) in, 179
ligaments in, 178
Little League elbow syndrome
   in, 180–181
medial epicondylitis (golfer's
   elbow) in, 179
movement of, 177
muscles of, 177–178
neuritis in, 181
olecranon in, 177, **178**, 182
questions and answers about,
   184–185
radius in, 177, **178**, 182
sprains in, 181–182
stiffness and pain in, 184
surgical treatment of, 181–183
ulna in, 177, **178**
ulnar nerve (funny bone) in,
   178, 181
Volkmann's ischemic
   contracture in, 183
Electrical stimulation (*See also*
   Transcutaneous electrical
   nerve stimulation), 148
Electrocoagulation, 158
Electrolytes, 3
Electromyogram (EMG), 134
Endorphins, 18
Epiphysis of shoulder, 170

Equilateral spiral, in hand,
   188–189
Erythrocyte sedimentation rate
   (*See also* Sedimentation
   rate tests), 70
Exercise, 25, 31–66, **171**
   active rest, 52
   activities as, 38–40
   aerobic, 32–33, 51–52, 58
   aging and, 32–34, 59, 61
   aids to, 49–51
   Alexander method, 56
   ankle, 108
   vs. arthritis, 17–18, 29
   balance, 40–42, 65–66
   benefits of, by age group, 58
   contraindications to, 58
   cross training, 54–55
   diet and, 61–62
   Eastern (Asian)-style, 55–56
   elbow, 179–180, 180
   equipment for, 57–58
   excuses for, 41–42, 58–50
   fat loss and, 34–36, 58
   Feldenkrais, 56
   fluid loss and, 34
   foot, 119, **119–120**
   hip, **76**, **77**
   illness vs., 33
   infants and children, 31,
      60–61
   isokinetic, 57
   isometric, 49, 51
   low-intensity/low-impact, 38
   metabolic vs. athletic fitness,
      59–60
   motivation for, 64–65
   myths about, 35–36
   natural or outdoor, 54
   neck, 133, 136
   oxygen utilization during, 59
   Pilates, 57
   pointers for good technique in,
      37

position sense (proprioception),
    48–49
prescription for, 38–40
Project PACE, 41
questions and answers about,
    57–66
resistance, 39–40
risk factors of, 60
scheduling, 36–37
shoulder, 167, **168–169**
special techniques in, 56–57
spine and back, 154, 162, 163
sports injuries and, 63–64
strength-building, 53, 54
stretching, 43–48
ultimate performance through,
    62–63
walking as, 50–51
warm up, 37
weight control and, 33–36, 62
weight training, 39, 50
winter conditioning, 63–64
women and, 53–54
wrist and hand, 197
Extension, 4
Extensor-supinator muscles,
    elbow, 177–178

Facets, vertebral facets, 141, **142,**
    143
Fascia, 11
Fasciitis, 11
Fat loss through exercise, 34–36,
    58
Fat pads, 6–7
Feet (*See* Foot)
Feldene (*See* piroxicam)
Feldenkrais exercises, 56
Femur, 67, **69**
Fibonnaci series, in describing
    hand configuration, 188
Fibrocartilage, 2, 99
Fibromyalgia, 159

Fibrositis, 11
Fibrous tissue, 1, 2, 10
Fibula, 105
Fingers (*See* Wrist and hand)
Flat foot (pes planus), 112–113,
    116–117, **116**
Flexion, 4
Flexor-pronator muscles, elbow,
    177–178
Fluid loss through exercise, 34
Foot, 4, 111–128
    anatomy and structure of,
        112–113, **112**
    arch of, 112
    arthritis in, 122, 124
    ballet and, 122, 127
    bones and ligaments of, 113,
        114, 127
    bunions (hallux valgus) and,
        121–123, 128
    bursitis in, 121
    calcaneal apophysitis (Sever's
        disease) in, 119
    calcaneus (heel bone) in, 117
    care of, 125
    clubfoot (congenital talipes
        equinovarus) in, 123–124
    corns and, 121
    deformity of, 115
    diabetes and, 117–118
    exercises for, 119, **119–120**
    flat foot condition (pes planus)
        in, 112–113, 116–117, **116**
    footwear and 113–117, 122,
        126–128
    fractures to, 117
    gout in, 124
    hallux rigidus of toe in, 123
    heel pain and injuries in, 117,
        119–121
    high arches in, 113, 116–117,
        116
    high heels and, 128
    joints in, 113

muscles of, 113
plantar fasciitis in, 119
questions and answers about,
    126–128
size of, 114–115
soft tissues complaints of, 117
soles of, 126
spurs in, 119
surgical treatment of, 121, 122,
    124
syndactyly (extra toes) on, 127
toe problems and, 121, 128
toe-walking gait in children
    and, 128
transverse arch collapse in, 123
walking and weight-bearing in,
    111, 113–114, 128
in women, 114–115, 127
Footwear, 113–117, 122, 126–128
Foramina, 130
Fractures and dislocations, 6
    ankle, 106–108
    elbow, 181, 182
    foot, 117
    neck, 131
    shoulder, 170–172
    spine and, 145–146, 163–164
    wrist and hand, 190–193
Frozen shoulder, 167–168
Function of joints, 1–2
Functional reserve, 40
"Funny bone" (See Ulnar nerve)
Fusion (See Arthrodesis)

Gamekeeper's thumb, 194
Ganglion cysts, 194
Gaucher's disease, 71
Genetic engineering, 63
Genetic therapy for rheumatoid
    arthritis, 23
Giant cell arthritis, 12
Glenohumeral joint, 165
Glenoid (shoulder socket), 165, 172

Glenoid labrum, 166
Gliding joint, 4, **5**
Gluck, Theophilus, 103
Glucosamine, glucosamine sul-
    fate, 17
Gold treatment, in rheumatoid
    arthritis, 22
Golfer's elbow, 11, 179
Gonorrhea, and arthritis, 11
Gout, gouty arthritis, **13**, 15,
    24–26, 28–29, 124
Grasp and grip, 187–188, 190,
    191
Guinea worm, and arthritis, 11

Hallux rigidus of toe, 123
Hallux valgus (bunions), 121–123
Hammertoes, 121, 122, 128
Hamstrings, 90
Hand (See Wrist and hand), 187
Hansen's disease and arthritis, 11
Headache, 12, 129, 132
Heat therapy 18, 132, 136
Heberden's nodes, 14
Heel pain and injuries, 117,
    119–121
Hemorrhagic joint disease, 28
Herbal remedies, osteoarthritis, 19
Herniated discs, 134, 146,
    150–154, **151**, 157, 158
Heterotopic ossification, 83–84,
Hinge joint, 4, **5**, 177
Hip, 4, 12, 21, 67–85, **69**, 166
    acetabulum in, 67, **69**, 67
    in adults, 73–83
    arthritis in, 75–83
    arthrodesis (fusion) surgery
        for, 78
    bursitis in, 73–74
    fractures in, 74–75
    osteotomy and, 78
    "snapping hip" in, 74
    tendinitis in, 74

total joint replacement in,
78–80, **81**, **82**
arthritis in, 70, 75–83
arthrodesis (fusion) surgery
for, 78
aseptic necrosis in, 85
avascular necrosis in, 71, 72
ball-and-socket of, 67
blood supply to, 70
bone cement and, in replacement surgery, 84
in children, 69–73
avascular necrosis in, 71, 72
congenital dislocation in, 84
degenerative arthritis in, 70
delayed diagnosis of, 70
developmental hip dysplasia
(DDH) in, 71–72
factors contributing to, 69–70
infection and, 70, 71
Legg-Calvé-Perthes (LCP) disease in, 72–73
slipped capital femoral epiphysis in, 73
transient synovitis in, 71
workup and history of illness
for, 70
congenital dislocation in, 84
developmental hip dysplasia
(DDH) in, 71–72
dislocation of, congenital, 14
exercises for, **76–77**
femur in, 67, **69**
fractures in, 74–75
heterotopic ossification in, 83–84
infection in, 70, 71
joint capsule of, 69
Legg-Calvé-Perthes (LCP)
disease in, 72–73
lever action of, 67–68, **68**
ligaments of, 68
ligamentum teres of, 68
lubrication of, 69
muscles of, 67, 69

myositis ossificans in, 84
obturator nerve for, 70
osteotomy and, 78
pelvis and, **69**
physical therapy and, 75
proximal femoral focal
deficiency in, 84
questions and answers about,
83–85
slipped capital femoral
epiphysis in, 73
"snapping hip" in, 74
synovial membrane of, 69
tendinitis in, 74
total joint replacement in,
78–80, **81**, **82**
transient synovitis in, 71
trochanter in, 69
tumors in, 83
Housemaid's knee, 11, 94
Human growth factor, 204
Humeroradial joints, 177
Humeroulnar joint, 177
Humerus, 165, 170, 177, **178**,
182
Hunchback (*See* kyphosis)
Hyaline cartilage, 2, 6, 9, 99
Hyaluronate (Hyalgan), 17
Hydroxychloroquine, 22
Hyperlordosis (*See also* lordosis),
146
Hypothyroidism, 14
Hysterical back pain, 146

Ibuprofen (Motrin), 16
Immovable joints, 2, 4
Immunosuppressive drugs, 22
Indomethacin (Indocin), 16
Infections (osteomylelitis), 11, 28,
70, 71, 95, 102, 193, 204
Infections arthritis, 11, 28
Inflammatory arthritis (*See*
Rheumatoid arthritis)

Inflammatory response and
arthritis, 10–11, 204
Interferon, 22
Intervertebral discs, 142–143,
142, 145
Intra-articular fractures, 192
Intradiscal electrothermal therapy
(IDET), 163
Intravenous immune gamma
globulin (IgG), 22
Invertebrates, 1
Isokinetic exercises, 57
Isometric exercises, 49, 51

Jaw, 12
Joint, defined, 1
Joint capsule (*See* Capsule)
Joint cavity, 3
Joint replacement surgery, 23,
78–80, **81, 82**, 97–98,
102–103, 183
Joint space, **2**
Jumper's knee, 11
Juvenile rheumatoid arthritis, 21

Kienböck's disease, 200–201
Knee, 2, 4, 6, 20, 21, **48**, 87–103
anatomy of, 88, **89**
arthritis and, 10, 88, 97–98,
102, 103
arthrodesis (fusion surgery) in,
99
Baker's cyst in, 94, 96–97
bowleg (genu varum) condition
in, 95, 102, 113
braces for, 102
bursitis in, 94
cartilage in, 99
chondromalacia patellae in, 96
deformity of, 95–97
diagnosis of disorders in,
93–94

disuse atrophy or wasting of
muscles in, 90–93
exercises for, 90–93, **91–93**, 100
fibrocartilage vs. hyaline cartilage in, 99
hamstrings and, 90
infections (osteomyelitis) in, 95
injuries and trauma to, 87–89,
95, 99–100
joint replacement surgery in,
97–98, 102–103
kneecap removal and, 102
knock-knee (genu valgum)
condition in, 95, 102, 113
ligaments of, 87, 88–89,
100–101
malignancies (osteogenic
sarcoma) in, 95
meniscal lesions or injury in,
96, 100, 101–102
muscle strength and, 90–93
nerves of, and pain, 99
Osgood-Schlatter disease in, 95
osteoarthritis of, 48
osteochondritis dissecans in, 95
osteonecrosis in, 14
patellar subluxation or
dislocation in, 96
pathologic synovial plicae in,
100
pathology of, 94–97
popliteal cysts in, 96–97
questions and answers about,
98–103
rehabilitation of, following
injury/surgery, 101
semilunar cartilages or minisci,
88, 96, 100, 101
surgical treatment (arthroscopic
and reconstructive) of, 87,
89–90, 94, 96, 97, 100–101,
102
symptoms of inflammation in,
87–88

torn meniscus in, 96, 100,
    101–102
unicompartmental arthroplasty
    for, 97
walking and, 88
weight-bearing ability of, 98
Kneecap removal, 102
Knock-knee (genu valgum), 95,
    102, 113
Kyphoplasty, 163–164
Kyphosis (hunchback), 144, 146

Lamina of vertebrae, 140
Laser treatments, 204
Lateral epicondylitis (tennis
    elbow), 179
Legg-Calvé-Perthes (LCP)
    disease, 72–73
Lenox Hill brace, 102
Leprosy and arthritis, 11
Lever action of joints,67–68, **68**
Lévy, Janine, 31
Ligamentitis, 11
Ligaments, 1, **2**, 3, 11
    in ankle, 105
    in elbow, 178
    in foot, 113, 114
    in hip, 68
    in knee, 87, 88–89, 100–101
    in neck, 130
    in shoulder, 167
    in spine, 141–142
    in wrist and hand, 189, **189**,
        193–196
Ligamentum teres of hip, 68
Limb joints, 3, 4
Liniments, 17
Little League elbow syndrome,
    180–181
Little League shoulder syndrome,
    170
Loading conditions, 2
Local pain, 134

Locked joints, 6
Longitudinal arch of hand, 188
Lordosis (swayback), 144, 146
Low-intensity/low-impact
    exercises, 38
Lubrication of joints, 1, 3, 6, 10,
    69
Lumbar vertebrae, 140, **141**, 143
Lupus, 29, 71
Lyme disease, 29

Magnet treatments, 18–19
Magnetic resonance imaging
    (MRI), 70, 94, 134, 145, 154
Malignancies (osteogenic
    sarcoma) (*See also* Tumors),
    95
Mallet finger, 194
Mallet toe, 121
Marcher's heel, 11
Massage, 132
Mating pairs of joint surfaces, 4
Mechanics of joints, 4–6
Medial epicondylitis (golfer's
    elbow), 179
Medications for arthritis, 14–20,
    22–23
Meniscal lesions or injury, knee,
    96, 100, 101
Menisci, 3
Mesoderm, in formation of bone
    and joints, 3
Metabolic vs. athletic fitness,
    59–60
Metacarpals, 188, **189**, 192, 194
Metatarsal arch, 112
Metatarsalgia, 128
Methotrexate, 22
Microdecompression surgery, 203
Mitochondria, 63
Motrin (*See* Ibuprofen)
Mucocutaneous lesions, 27
Muscle relaxants, 17

Muscle spasm, in neck and, 134
Muscles, 3, 11, 14
    aging and, 32–34
    in elbow, 177–178
    in foot, 113
    in hip, 67, 69
    in knee and, 90–93
    in neck, 130–131
    in shoulder, 165–166
    in wrist and hand, 188, 189,
        189, **190**
Myalgia, 11
Mycoplasma bacteria and
        arthritis, 11
Myelogram, 158
Myositis, 11, 84

Nabumetone (Relafen), 16
Naproxen (Naprosyn), 16
Natural/outdoor exercise, 54
Neck, 129–138
    abnormalities of, 132
    in adults, 132–137
    anatomy of, 130, **131**
    arthritis in, 131
    care of, 138
    cervical joint lock in, 135–136
    in children, 131–132
    diseases in, 131
    exercises for, 133, 136
    foramina of, 130
    fractures and dislocations of,
        131
    headache and, 129, 132
    herniated disc and, 134
    injuries to, 131, 132
    ligaments and muscles of,
        130–131
    movement in, 130–131
    muscle spasm in, 134
    nerves in, 130
    occipital bone of skull and, 130
    pain in, 129–135

pinched nerve in, 134
posture and, 133, 134
questions and answers about,
    137–138
slipped discs in, 138
spinal cord and, 130
torticollis (wry neck, stiff neck)
    in, 131–132, 135, 137–138
vertebrae of, 129, 130
whiplash injury to, 132–133
Neoplasms, 83
Nerve conduction velocity (NCV)
    tests, 134
Nerve root pain, 135
Neuritis, in elbow, 181
Neuropathic joints, diabetes and,
    110
Nonsteroidal antiinflammatory
    drugs (NSAIDs), 15–16, 26,
    74, 75, 132, 157, 170, 179,
    181, 196
Novocaine, 74

Obstetrical palsy of shoulder, 175
Obturator nerve, hip, 70
Occipital bone of skull, 130
Occupational therapists, 23
Olecranon, 177, **178**, 182
Opposition of thumb, 189–190,
    190
Orthopaedic surgeons, 23
Osgood-Schlatter disease, 95
Ossification, 3
Osteoarthritis (*See* Arthritis,
    osteo-)
Osteochondral autograft of knee
    cartilage, 90
Osteochondral dysplasia, 102
Osteochondral grafting, 20
Osteochondritis dissecans, 95, 108
Osteonecrosis, 14
Osteotomy, 78
Oxaprozin (Daypro), 16

Pac Man tendinitis, 11
Pain
    of arthritis, 10, 11–12, 21, 22
    neck, 129, 131–132, 134–135
    in spine, 145, 154–159, 154
Pain fibers, to knee, 99
Palliative vs. curative treat-
    ments, 19
Pannus of rheumatoid arthritis,
    21
Parasitic infection and arthritis,
    11
Patellar subluxation or disloca-
    tion, 96
Pathologic synovial plicae, knee,
    100
Pedicles of vertebrae, 140
Pelvis, **69**
Penicillamine, 22
Perthes' disease, 71
Phalanges, 188, **189**, **190**, 192, 194
Physical therapy, 23, 75
Pigmented villondular synovitis,
    29–30
Pilates exercise, 57
Pillows, 132
Pinch grip, 187
Pinched nerve, neck, 134
Pinching injuries within joints,
    fat pad, 7
Piroxicam (Feldene), 16
Pivot joint, **5**
Plantar fasciitis, foot, 119
Podagra, in gouty arthritis, 24
Polydactyly (extra fingers), 127
Polymethyl methacrylate (bone
    cement), 84
Polymyalgia rheumatica, 12
Popliteal cysts, 96–97
Position sense (proprioception)
    and exercise, 48–49, 99
Posture, 133, 134, 143–145, 147,
    150
Power grip, 188, **191**

Precision grip, **191**
Project PACE, 41
Prolotherapy, 157
Proprioception, 48–49, 99
Prostaglandins, 16
Prostate, back pain and, 153
Prosthetics, 204
Protein, 3
Proximal femoral focal deficiency,
    84
Pseduogout, 28–29
Pseudarthrosis of clavicle, con-
    genital, 174
Psoriatic arthritis, 28
Psychogenic rheumatism, 12
Purine, in gouty arthritis, 25

Quadriceps muscles and knee,
    48–49, 90
Quiz on joint knowledge, 209–211

Radius, 177, **178**, 182, 187
Range-of-motion exercises, 17–18
Reactive arthritis, 27–28
Reduction of fractures, 72, 107
Referred pain, 131, 134–135
Reflex sympathetic dystrophy,
    197–198
Reiter's syndrome (*See* Reactive
    arthritis)
Relafen (*See* Nabumetone)
Remicade, 23
Repetitive strain syndrome,
    73–74, 195
Research on joint medicine,
    203–205
Resistance exercises, 39–40
Rheumatic fever vs. arthritis, 28
Rheumatism, 11–12
Rheumatoid arthritis (*See*
    Arthritis, rheumatoid)
Rheumatoid spolylitis, 146

Rheumatologists, 23
Rib facets, 140
Ribs, 4, 11, 144
RICE therapy for sprains, 106
Rickets, 102
Rofecoxib (Vioxx), 16
Rotation, 4
Rotator cuff, 166, 167

Sacroiliac joint dysfunction, 158
Sacrum, 140, **141**
Saddle joint, 4, **5**
Salicin (*See also* Aspirin), 15
Salmonella poisoning and
    arthritis, 29
Sarcopenia, 32
Scaphoid fractures, 192
Scapulothoracic joint, 165
Scheuermann's disease, 146
Sciatica, 14, 150–151, 154
Scoliosis, 144, 146–148, **147**
Sedimentation rate test, for
    arthritis, 12, 22, 70
Selenium, 61
Semilunar cartilages or minisci,
    knee, 88, 96, 100, 101
Separation injury in shoulder,
    170–171, 172
Sever's disease, 119
Shoes (*See* Footwear)
Shoulder, 2, 4, 14, 67, 165–175
    acromioclavicular joint in, 165,
        170–171
    acromion of, 166
    adhesive capsulitis or frozen,
        167–168, **171**
    anatomy of, 165–166, **166**
    arthritis in, 172–173, 174
    bursa and bursitis in,
        166–167
    clavicle and, 165, 170
    congenital pseudarthrosis of
        clavicle in, 174

epiphysis in, 170
exercise of, 167, **168–169**
exercises for, **171**
fractures and dislocations of,
    170–172
fusion in, 174
glenohumeral joint in, 165
glenoid (shoulder socket) in,
    165, 172
glenoid labrum in, 166
humerus and, 165, 170
injuries to, 166–170
ligaments in, 167
Little League shoulder syn-
    drome in, 170
movement of, 165
muscles and tendons in,
    165–166
nerves of, 173–174, 175
obstetrical palsy in, 175
questions and answers about,
    173–175
rotator cuff in, 166, 167
scapulothoracic joint in, 165
separation injury in, 170–171,
    172
shoulder pointer injury in, 170
slipping in, 172
sternum and, 165
stinger or burner injury in,
    173–174
subluxation of, voluntary or
    habitual, 174–175
surgical treatment of, 172, 174
thermal capsular shift for, 172
Shoulder pointer injury, 170
Sickle cell anemia, 71
Sjögren's syndrome, 28
Skeleton, 1
Skull joints, 3, 4
Sleep position, spine and,
    162–163
Slipped capital femoral epiphysis,
    73

Slipped or ruptured vertebral
discs, 138, 150–154, **151**
Slipping shoulder, 172
Smoking and health, 164
"Snapping hip," 74
Social workers, 23
Somatic referred pain, 135
Space boots, 121
Spinal cord, 130, 141
Spinal stenosis, 164
Spine, 12, 139–164
in adults, 148–159
anatomy of, 140–141, **141**
arthritis and, 146, 151, 164
artificial stainless steel disks
for, 203
bone grafts and fusion in, 148
braces for, 146
care of, **152**, **153**, 159
cartilage in, 144
cauda equina syndrome in, 158
causes of back injuries and
pain, 149–150
cervical vertebrae of, 140, **141**,
143
chemonucleolysis in, 158
in children, 145–148
coccyx of, 140
configuration and curvature of,
139–140, 143–144,
146–147
curvature (abnormal) of,
144–145, 146–148
disc growth in, using human
growth factor, 204
discitis in, 145
discs in, vertebral discs,
142–143, **142**, 145
electrocoagulation in, 158
exercises for, 154, 162, 163
fibromyalgia in, 159
fractures and dislocations in,
145–146, 163–164
fusion of, 157

herniated discs in, 146,
150–154, **151**, 157, 158
hyperlordosis in, 146
hysterical back pain in, 146
injuries to, 148–159
Internet addresses for information on, 159–161
intradiscal electrothermal
therapy (IDET) in, 163
kyphoplasty in, 163–164
kyphosis (hunchback) in, 144,
146
ligaments (ligamenta flava) of,
141–142
lordosis (swayback) in, 144,
146
lumbar vertebrae of, 140, **141**,
143
movement in, 141–142
myelogram of, 158
osteoid osteoma in, 146
pain in, 145, 154–159, 162
posture and, 143–145, 147, 150
prolotherapy in, 157
prostate and, 153
questions and answers about,
162–164
rheumatoid spolylitis in, 146
rib facets in, 140
ribs and, 144
sacroiliac joint dysfunction in,
158
sacrum of, 140, **141**
Scheuermann's disease in, 146
sciatica in, 150–151, 154
scoliosis in, 144, 146–148, **147**
sexual positions for lower back
pain in, **155–157**
sleep position and, 162–163
slipped or ruptured discs in,
150–154, **151**
smoking and health of, 164
spinal cord and, 141
spinal stenosis in, 164

spondylolisthesis in, 145–146, 153

spondylolysis, 146

sprains to, 150

in standing and walking, 143–144

steroid injections and, 157, 159

stress fracture in, 145–146

stress, tension, and muscle spasms in, 151–152

surgical treatment of, 146, 148, 151, 154, 157–158

synovial joints in, 143

thoracic vertebrae of, 140, **141**, 143, 144, 146

transcutaneous electrical nerve stimulation (TENS) in, 158

trigger points of pain in, 158–159

tumors in, 146, 153–154

vascular disease and, 154

vertebrae of, 139–141, **141**, **142**

vertebral facets, 141, **142**, 143

weight-bearing in, 149–150

Spondylitis Association of America, 27

Spondylolisthesis, 145–146, 153

Spondylolysis, 146

Sports injuries, 11, 63–64, 108–109, 170, 179, 180–181, 196

Sprains (*See also* Whiplash injury), 6, 106–107, 150, 181–182, 192, 193–194

Spurs, heel, 119

Stem cells and repair of injury, 204

Sternum, 11, 165

Steroids (*See* Corticosteroids)

Stiff neck (*See* Torticollis)

Stiffness of arthritis, 10, 12, 14–15, 21, 22

Still's disease (*See* Juvenile rheumatoid arthritis)

Stinger or burner shoulder injury, 173–174

Strength-building exercises, 53, 54

Stretching exercises, 43–48

Subluxation of shoulder, voluntary or habitual, 174–175

Sulindac (Clinoril), 16

Surgical treatments

amputation in, 204

in ankle, 107–108

arthroscopic surgery in, 203

computer-generated imagery in, 205

computerized operative planning for, 204

in elbow, 181, 182, 183

in foot, 121, 122, 124

in knee, 87, 89–90, 94, 96, 97, 100–101, 102

microdecompression, 203

in osteoarthritis, 19–20

in rheumatoid arthritis, 23

in shoulder, 172, 174

in spine, 146, 148, 151, 154, 157–158

transplantation of joints in, 204

Swayback (*See* Lordosis)

Swelling of arthritis, 10, 21, 22

Synarthroses, 4

Syndactyly (extra toes), 127

Synovectomy, 23, 29–30

Synovial articulations, 4

Synovial fluid, 6, 10, 15

Synovial joints, 6, 143

Synovial lining/membrane, **2**, 3, 21, 69

Synovial plicae, pathologic, knee, 100

Synovitis, 71

Tae-bo/tai-chi, 55–56

Talus bones of foot, 105

Temporomandibular joint, 29
Tendinitis, 11, 74
Tendons, 3, 11, **189**, **190**, 194, 199
Tennis elbow, 11, 179
Thermal capsular shift, 172
Thermography, 196
Thixotropy of synovial fluid, 6
Thoracic vertebrae, 140, **141**, 143, 144, 146
Thumb (*See* Wrist and hand)
Tibia, 105
Toes, 24, 121
Tolmetin (Tolectin), 16
Topical treatments for osteoarthritis, 17
Torn meniscus, knee, 96
Torticollis, neck, 131–132, 135, 137–138
Total joint replacement, hip, 78–80, **81**, **82**
Toxins, in rheumatoid arthritis, 21
Traction, 72, 132, 135, 157
Transcutaneous electrical nerve stimulation (TENS), 18, 132, 158
Transient synovitis, 71
Transition grip, **191**
Transplantation of joints, 204
Transverse arch collapse, in foot, 123
Transverse arch of hand, 188
Transverse volar carpal ligament, 195–196
Trigger points of pain in spine, 158–159
Trochanter, 69
Tuberculosis, and arthritis, 11
Tumors, 83, 146, 153–154, 204
Types of joints, 3–4

Ulna, 177, **178**, 187
Ulnar nerve (funny bone), 178, 181

Ultrasound treatments, 18, 70, 179–180
Unicompartmental arthroplasty, 97
Urethritis, 27
Uric acid, in gouty arthritis, 15, 24, 124

Vascular disease and back pain, 154
Verneuil, 103
Vertebrae (*See also* Neck; Spine), 129, 130, 140, 139–141, **141**, **142**
Vertebral discs, 142–143, **142**, 145
Vertebral facets, 141, **142**, 143, 141
Vertebral joints, 3, 4
Vertebrates, 1
Vioxx (*See* Rofecoxib)
Viral arthritis, 11
Visceral disturbances, 12
Visceral referred pain, 135
Viscosupplementation, in arthritis treatment, 17
Vitamin B complex, 61
Vitamin C, 16, 61
Vitamin D, 16, 102
Vitamin E, 16, 61
Vitamin therapy for arthritis, 16
Volkmann's ischemic contracture, 183
Voltaren (*See* Diclofenate sodium)

Walking as exercise, 38–39, 50–51
Warm-up exercises, 37
Weaver's bottom, 11
Weeping lubrication, 10
Weight-bearing joints, 2, 14, 21
Weight control, 17, 26, 33–36, 62
Weight training exercises, 39, 50

Whiplash injury, 6, 132–133
Winter conditioning exercises,
  63–64
Women and exercise, 53–54
Women's Sports Foundation, The,
  54
Wrist and hand, 4, 14, 21, 187–201
  anatomy of, 188–189, **189**, **190**
  arthritis in, 193, 194–195
  athletic injury to, 196
  Bennett's fracture in, 192
  bleeding injuries in, 198–199
  bones of, 187, 188
  boxer's fracture in, 192–193
  carpal tunnel in, 188, 195–196
  carpal tunnel syndrome in,
    195–196
  carpals of, **189**
  close-packed position of, 6
  club hand deformity in, 200
  Colles fracture in, 190, 192
  de Quervain's disease in, 199
  deformities in, 21, 199
  Dupuytren's contracture in, 199
  equilateral spiral in, 188–189
  exercise for, 197
  first aid for, 198–199
  fractures in, 190–193
  function of, 189–190, **191**
  gamekeeper's thumb in, 194
  ganglion cysts in, 194
  grasp and grip in, 187–188,
    190, **191**
  infections in, 193
  injuries to, 199–200
  intra-articular fractures in, 192
  Kienböck's disease in, 200–201
  ligaments of, 189, **189**,
    193–196

longitudinal arch of hand in,
  188
mallet finger in, 194
metacarpals in, 188, **189**, 192,
  194
movement of, 187, 189
muscles of, 188, 189, **189**, **190**
opposition of thumb in,
  189–190, **190**
phalanges in, 188, **189**, **190**,
  192, 194
polydactyly (extra fingers) and,
  127
questions and answers about,
  198–201
radius and, 187
reflex sympathetic dystrophy
  in, 197–198
repetitive strain syndrome in,
  195
scaphoid fractures in, 192
soft tissue injuries to, 190
sprains in, 192, 193–194
tendons of, **189**, **190**, 194, 199
therapy and rehabilitation in,
  200
transverse arch of hand in, 188
transverse volar carpal ligament in, 195–196
ulna and, 187
Wry neck (*See* Torticollis)

X-rays, 15, 22, 94, 134, 135, 138,
  145, 154, 158, 179

Yoga, 56